## IS KAVA THE ANSWER FOR YOU?

- Do you feel tense at the end of your work day?

- Do you worry excessively?

- Are you edgy and irritable?

- Do you have trouble sleeping?

- Is it sometimes difficult to focus?

- Do you experience periods of anxiety for no specific reason?

- Do your muscles ache much of the time?

- Do you long for the ability to just relax?

# KAVA

## Nature's Stress Relief

**KATHRYN M. CONNOR, M.D.**
**and Donald S. Vaughan**

A CMD PUBLISHING BOOK

AVON BOOKS NEW YORK

The ideas, procedures, and suggestions in this book are intended to supplement, not replace, the medical advice of a trained medical professional. All matters regarding your health require medical supervision. Consult your physician before adopting the suggestions in this book, as well as about any condition that may require diagnosis or medical attention. The author and publisher disclaim any liability arising directly or indirectly from the use of this book.

AVON BOOKS, INC.
1350 Avenue of the Americas
New York, New York 10019

Copyright © 1999 by CMD Publishing, a division of Current Medical Directions, Inc.
Illustration by Patricia Shea
Published by arrangement with CMD Publishing, a division of Current Medical Directions, Inc.
ISBN: 0-380-80641-X
www.avonbooks.com

First Avon Books Printing: March 1999

AVON TRADEMARK REG. U.S. PAT. OFF. AND IN OTHER COUNTRIES, MARCA REGISTRADA, HECHO EN U.S.A.

Printed in the U.S.A.

WCD 10 9 8 7 6 5 4 3 2

# CONTENTS

# ONE

~~~~~~~

## *What Is Kava?*

**FACT:** Kava has been consumed as a medicinal and recreational herb by the natives of the South Pacific islands for thousands of years.

**FACT:** Kava is taking the United States and the world by storm and promises to equal St. John's Wort, gingko biloba, and echinacea in popularity.

**FACT:** Kava can ease anxiety and induce sound sleep as effectively as many prescription anxiety-reducing medications and sedatives—at a fraction of the cost.

**FACT:** Kava has many other potential medical applications, including use as an anti-inflammatory, diuretic, analgesic, and bronchial agent.

**FACT:** Kava has minimal side effects and is safe when consumed in moderation.

~~~~~~~

*Meet Betty. She's 33, single, and a midlevel manager for a company that manufactures children's shoes. Betty has had One of Those Days, the kind that start badly and only get worse. Her alarm clock didn't go off, so she was 15 minutes late for work. Her boss, already in an ugly mood, loudly reprimanded Betty for her tardiness in front of the entire office, then stacked her desk with reports that absolutely had to be completed before the end of the business day. Eager to please—and to keep her job—Betty locked herself in her office and skipped lunch to get the work done, only to be told at 4:55 that half of the reports were no longer needed. On the way home, she was splashed with mud, nearly run over by an errant taxi, and barked at by a neighbor's nasty Doberman.*

*By the time Betty unlocked the door to her small apartment she was a quivering, crying mass of stress and anxiety. Her head throbbed, her shoulders ached, and her stomach burned from hunger and frustration. In the past, Betty would have dealt with this terrible day by downing a couple of prescription tranquilizers and zoning out in front of the television. But in an attempt to better her life, Betty now avoids most commercial medications in favor of more natural remedies. On this hectic and miserable day, for example, Betty relieves her stress, anxiety, and pending insomnia with two piping hot cups of kava tea sweetened with honey, followed by a healthy meal of pasta, green salad, and fruit juice.*

Betty is not alone in her appreciation of the amazing herbal calmative known as kava. Indigenous to the islands of the South Pacific, kava is rapidly becoming one of the most popular medicinal herbs in the world. According to a report in the *Wall Street Journal*, US sales of kava via food stores, drugstores, and mass merchandisers topped an impressive $2.95 million in 1997, and importers say the sky's the limit as more and more people are turned on to the herb's astounding ability to gently relieve stress and anxiety and ensure a good night's sleep with virtually none of the side effects commonly associated with prescription and over-the-counter medications. The skyrocketing popularity of kava is just a small part of an ongoing global shift from synthetic medications to herbal remedies for the treatment of a wide range of medical conditions such as mild depression (St. John's Wort), memory impairment (ginkgo biloba), and seasonal colds (echinacea).

If you've never heard of kava, don't feel bad. Until relatively recently, it was one of the world's best-kept herbal secrets, known only to the residents of the South Pacific islands and a few lucky westerners who consumed the herb with the natives in time-honored ceremonies or at public "kava bars." But word is out and spreading quickly regarding kava's many therapeutic applications, some of which are so effective that many health-care professionals have started recommending it to patients afflicted with stress, anxiety, insomnia, and other complaints. In this introductory chapter, we'll discuss the history of kava, its traditional uses, and its botany.

## What is kava?

Kava, known scientifically as *Piper methysticum*, is a member of the pepper tree family. It is also the name of the beverage prepared from the plant's root. Kava is common to Oceania—the South Pacific island regions of Polynesia, Melanesia, and Micronesia that include Fiji, Samoa, Tonga, and Tahiti—and has a long history of cultural, social, and therapeutic applications. In recent years, kava has also gained popularity among the natives of Hawaii, New Guinea, and Australia, where it is used for both medicinal and recreational purposes.

Kava goes by many names. Depending on the region, it may be known as kava-kava, awa, waka, lawena, sakau, yaqona, or yanggona. But to paraphrase Shakespeare, kava by any other name is still kava. The exact origin of the plant is unknown, although most botanists believe it originated in northern Vanuatu, a small chain in the Solomon Islands.

## What does kava look like?

Kava is a perennial shrub that typically grows from three to ten feet tall and occasionally higher. It has smooth,

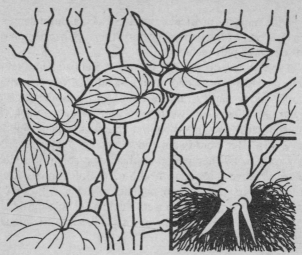

The kava plant's leaves and stems. *Inset:* the rhizome (root), which is harvested to make kava products.

pointed, heart-shaped leaves, a soft-wooded stem and a rhizome (a root, or creeping stem) with a knotty crown that can grow up to nine feet long. It is the rhizome that is typically harvested, although other parts of the plant are occasionally used for various purposes. The shrub bears a small, narrow flower that looks like a yellow-green spike.

Kava prefers low elevations, constant moisture, and partial sun, which explains why it does so well in the South Pacific islands. It's a hearty plant that thrives best in rich soil, but it can also be found growing in rocky, less hospitable terrain. It is usually harvested when the plant is three or more years old and six to eight feet in height because that is when the therapeutic components of the root—known scientifically as kavalactones—are at their strongest.

## Can I buy kava seeds so I can plant my own?

No, kava doesn't bear seeds. In its native South Pacific territory, kava is cultivated much like sugarcane; sections of stalk are laid horizontally in mud trenches until they sprout, and then they are transplanted and allowed to grow to maturity. New stalks continually spring forth as the root grows, so the plant can reproduce itself for many, many years. Dozens of varieties of kava have been identified in various regions. Potency may vary from one variety to another, but the medicinal and physiological effects are essentially the same. Kava grows wild in most regions of the South Pacific, but most users prefer cultivated kava because it tends to be stronger and more effective.

### How long has kava been cultivated and used by the natives of the South Pacific islands?

Researchers are unsure, but archeological studies suggest the herb has been in widespread use for hundreds and probably thousands of years. The first westerners to report on the existence and use of kava were with British explorer Captain James Cook, who visited the South Pacific islands between 1768 and 1771 and called the plant "intoxicating pepper." Johann George Forster, a naturalist who accompanied Cook, published the first description of kava's various effects in 1777. Many researchers believe Cook was the first westerner to partake of the beverage made from the kava root, possibly during a tribal ceremony to greet the visiting foreigners. Intrigued, Cook brought kava back with him and introduced the herb to western civilization. Years later, the botanical was given its scientific name, *Piper methysticum* (the prefix *methy* is the Greek word for wine). Like the Native Americans, the Polynesians did not know how to ferment alcohol from fruit or grain prior to contact with Europeans. But kava extract, made by steeping ground root in coconut milk or cold water, was undoubtedly a safer and more therapeutic substitute.

### What do the natives of the South Pacific islands traditionally use kava for?

Kava has played, and continues to play, an integral role in almost every aspect of the lives of the South Pacific islanders. Historically, it was most commonly used during religious and cultural ceremonies. For example, drinking kava was an important gesture of goodwill when local natives greeted visiting dignitaries. President Lyndon Johnson and his wife, Lady Bird, were served kava during a trip to Samoa in 1965, and Pope John Paul II was given a cup of the beverage during a visit to Fiji in 1986. More recently, First Lady Hillary Rodham Clinton partook in this tradition while touring various regions of the South Pacific islands. Understandably, kava's cultural role in the South Pacific has been compared to that of wine in many parts of Europe, such as France and Italy.

Kava is a very social drink. Consumption tends to make users friendlier and more open to conversation. As a result, kava is often used as a pleasant, nonviolent way to settle disputes and arguments between neighbors and spouses. Some people believe the widespread use of kava could change global diplomacy for the better. In his 1937 book *Savage Civilization*, writer Tom Harrisson said of kava: "Your head is affected most pleasantly. Thoughts come cleanly. You feel friendly; not beer sentimental; never cross. The world gains no new color or rose tint; it fits in its pieces and is one (easily understandable) whole. You cannot hate with kava in you, and so it is used in the making up of quarrels, and in peacemaking. It would change the face of Geneva."

In some South Pacific cultures, the consumption of kava was strictly ritualized and the first bowl often went to the village chieftain or other high-ranking village member or visiting dignitaries. Today, kava is a beverage readily enjoyed by everyone regardless of class or social order, and in some regions kava bars, known as nakamals, greatly outnumber bars that serve alcohol. Because it induces a sense of calm and conviviality, many Polynesians enjoy getting together after a hard day at work and downing a few bowls of kava with friends and family. A sense of friendly familiarity takes over as the herb takes effect and it's not uncommon for minor acquaintances to quickly become good friends as lively conversation flows.

Kava has a great many other traditional uses. It is often consumed during important business meetings because it induces a sense of cooperation without affecting clarity of thought, and travelers frequently down a bowl or two before going on a long journey to make the trip a little easier to bear. Social occasions such as weddings, funerals, and birthdays are almost always celebrated with kava, and both the plant and the beverage are commonly offered as gifts of friendship.

## Is kava used medicinally by the South Pacific islanders?

Most definitely. Kava has a long history among the Polynesians as a medicinal herb and has long been used to ease stress and anxiety, induce a good night's sleep, ease minor aches and pains (users say it's just as effective as aspirin or acetaminophen), and restore vigor.

Because kava has effective diuretic and anti-inflammatory properties, it was also used to treat more serious medical problems including urinary tract infections, premenstrual syndrome, migraine headache, cystitis, gout, arthritis, digestive problems, whooping cough in children, and the symptoms of bronchial disorders such as asthma and tuberculosis. Some islanders also considered it a mild aphrodisiac because it relaxes the body while sharpening the senses.

Applied topically, kava was used to treat disorders ranging from fungal infections and painful insect stings to skin problems. There is also some anecdotal evidence that kava can prevent and even cure gonorrhea, although there is little scientific research to date to verify this action.

The kava root is the part of the plant most commonly used for therapeutic applications, although many Pacific islanders traditionally use the plant's stems, leaves, and bark for medicinal purposes including the treatment of chills, cold, headache, and general fatigue. One favorite island folk remedy recommends chewing a small amount of leaf buds and then giving the mash to a feverish or restless child to induce sleep. This technique may also be used to ease teething pain.

Although kava has been studied by westerners since the 1800s, only now are researchers starting to understand how it works and on what conditions it is most effective. Some uses have been solidly substantiated, such as easing stress and anxiety. Others are still in the research stage and have yet to be confirmed. Kava certainly isn't a cure-all—no herb is—but it looks like we've only touched the tip of the iceberg when it comes to the plant's medicinal potential.

## How was kava traditionally prepared?

To be honest, it's a pretty unpleasant story. Kava is a tough root and must be mashed pretty well before being added to coconut milk or cool water to create a beverage. In the past, islanders would chew the root until it was a pulpy consistency, then spit it into a large communal bowl. At one time the job was relegated to young boys and girls because they supposedly had the best teeth and strongest jaws. This was important because chewing kava was a grueling chore that was detested by pretty much everyone who had to do it. When there was sufficient root to make enough kava for all involved, water was added and the mixture was stirred until it had a muddy or dirty color, and then it was strained and served. Not surprisingly, Captain Cook and his crew were disgusted by the ritual when they first witnessed it; they considered it filthy and barbaric.

Today most kava root is prepared by hand or machine, especially at kava bars where large quantities are consumed daily. Chewing, or mastication, continues in only a few small areas, most notably the southern islands of Vanuatu and parts of Papua New Guinea, because many of the natives there believe mastication produces a more potent brew. Researchers say they may be right; studies suggest that chewing releases more kavalactones (the therapeutic components of the root) than hand or machine processing because saliva contains enzymes that break down the pulp.

## Was kava prepared any other way?

No. The preparation of kava was steeped in tradition and ritual, but the bottom line was that grinding the root (either by mouth, hand, or machine) and steeping it in cold water was the most effective way to make the strongest elixir. Cooking, boiling, or distilling kava root produced an inferior beverage and was seldom attempted.

## What does kava taste like?

Let's just say it isn't good. Kava tends to be quite sour and foul-tasting (the Hawaiian word for the herb—awa— means bitter) and is definitely an acquired taste. First-timers have used phrases such as "dirty sock water" and "totally gross" to describe their first bowl of kava—which explains why it is usually gulped rather than sipped. Good quality kava produces a temporary numbing of the tongue and mouth, but this does little to alleviate the awful taste. Kava can be sweetened with coconut milk or honey to make it a bit more palatable, but most kava connoisseurs prefer their kava straight. Kava tablets and capsules are available for those who don't want to go to the trouble of making the kava brew or who simply can't tolerate the taste. See Chapter 7: Shopping for Kava for more information on the various forms of kava and where to buy them.

## What's it like at a traditional South Pacific kava bar, or nakamal? Is it like visiting a nightclub or pub that serves alcohol?

Yes and no. They are similar in that people gather to drink and socialize, but the atmosphere at a nakamal is usually much quieter and low-key, the result of the calming effect of the kava itself. Most kava bars are simple structures made of bamboo, wood, scrap metal, or any other building materials that happen to be lying around. The floor is usually made of dirt, which is good because kava connoisseurs often spit a lot in an attempt to get rid of the bitter taste. A wood counter may serve as the bar, with benches ringing the outer walls and additional benches and chairs outside. Lighting is typically as simple as the structures themselves, and usually consists only of a kerosene lamp or a bare light bulb. Kava bars aren't known for their atmosphere; their main purpose is for social gathering.

The proprietor spends the late afternoon preparing the evening's kava in a large tub, using a machine to grind the root. The majority of kava bars don't open until sunset, when the locals return home from work tired and in need of soothing refreshment. Most prefer to enjoy kava before a meal because it is believed that the herb's effects are enhanced on an empty stomach. The equivalent of a dollar or so will get you a half coconut shell or cup of kava, which is usually downed in one gulp. After a serving or two, patrons visit with friends as the soothing effects of the herb take effect. Additional cups of kava may be consumed over the course of the evening, although two or three is the limit for most people. Most kava bars are open only a few hours each evening, after which the majority of patrons have consumed their fill and returned home for dinner.

There's another dramatic difference between kava bars and those that serve alcohol: Brawls are extremely rare at kava bars. The beverage promotes friendly conversation rather than fisticuffs, and most users find themselves too relaxed and tranquil to do anything more than chat.

**I've never consumed kava, but it sounds like fun. Before I run to my local health food store and buy some, can you tell me what I should expect?**

We have to answer that question in general terms because people tend to have a unique and individual response to kava, just as they do when they drink alcohol or consume any other body- or mind-altering substance. In addition, the varying quality of commercial kava products available in the United States and the different forms in which it can be consumed (pill, capsule, or tincture, for example) makes it difficult to detail exactly what one should expect.

In most cases, however, the effects of kava begin within an hour of consumption, and last four or more hours. People who are tense, nervous or anxious will notice the effects of the herb more dramatically than people who are already calm and relaxed. The range of sensations experienced by kava users is dramatic, but the most common include a sense of relaxation and general well-being, a feeling of contentment and/or mild euphoria, improved concentration and mental alertness, and a desire to be more sociable. The latter reaction is why kava is traditionally consumed in groups; it makes conversation easier and more fun. In addition, some users report a sense of sleepiness, while others say they feel more energized—at least temporarily. In most cases, alertness is followed hours later by a sedative effect.

Lewis Lewin, a prominent researcher of psychoactive drugs, wrote of the effects of kava consumption rather succinctly in a paper published in 1886 by the Berlin Medical Society: "A well prepared kava potion drunk in small quantities produces only pleasant changes in behavior. It is therefore a slightly stimulating drink which helps relieve great fatigue. It relaxes the body after strenuous efforts, clarifies the mind and sharpens the mental faculties. If a certain quantity of these active elements is absorbed they produce special narcotic effects."

Years later, in his book *Phantastica: Narcotic and Stimulating Drugs*, Lewin wrote further about kava: "When the mixture is not too strong, the subject attains a state of happy unconcern, well-being and contentment, free of physical or psychological excitement. At the beginning conversation comes in a gentle, easy flow and hearing and sight are honed, becoming able to perceive subtle shades of sound and vision. Kava soothes temperaments. The drinker never becomes angry, unpleasant, quarrelsome, or noisy, as happens with alcohol. Both natives and whites consider kava as a means of easing moral discomfort. The drinker remains master of his conscience and his reason."

## Can other parts of the kava plant produce the same effects as the root when consumed?

The stems and leaves of the kava plant contain kavalactones, but researchers know very little about their psychoactive properties; most studies of the herb involve root extract. South Pacific islanders have been known to make medicinal use of other parts of the kava plant, but the kava beverage is made almost exclusively from the root.

## Is kava unique in its widespread cultural use? Are the Polynesians the only people to show such devotion to a natural, mind-altering substance?

Not at all. Anthropologists tell us that almost every society, ancient or contemporary, has its favorite herbs or compounds—some more mind-altering than others. (Remember: While kava has mild anesthetic properties and can induce pleasant changes in mood and demeanor, relax muscles, reduce anxiety, and boost friendliness, it does not dramatically affect brain function nor is it addictive or otherwise dangerous when consumed in recommended quantities.) For example, natives of Southeast Asia get a rush from chewing betel nuts, while many members of the South American Andean culture get a similar high munching on coca leaves. The Mexican Huichol use peyote, and certain tribes in Africa smoke cannabis (marijuana) both for recreation and for religious reasons. In the United States, it could be said that alcohol, caffeine, and nicotine are our (legal) drugs of choice, although a great many Americans also consume their share of so-called recreational mind-altering drugs, most notably marijuana. Kava is unique in that it makes us feel good without impairing mental clarity or causing any serious side effects.

## Was the use of kava accepted by the early missionaries who tried to convert the natives of the South Pacific islands?

Tolerance for the use of kava varied. Anglican and Catholic priests were relatively accepting of kava and even drank it on occasion with the natives, but the early Protestant missionaries, who arrived in the late 1800s and early 1900s, were horrified by kava and did everything in their power to stop the natives from drinking it. The missionaries were repulsed by the way the beverage was made (many said chewing the plant made the resulting beverage a "devil's drink") and they considered kava a heathen elixir that had to be banished at all costs.

The methods of its manufacture aside, most missionaries didn't like kava because they compared its effects (erroneously) with those of alcohol. To them, a drunk was a drunk regardless of whether the person was inebriated on whiskey or merely pleasantly buzzed on kava. Most missionaries banned the use of kava among their members and among the natives they were trying to convert, forcing many into a sort of "kava underground." On some islands kava drinkers and manufacturers were harassed and even arrested merely for enjoying the traditional beverage. Others were ostracized and prohibited from attending church which, in retrospect, seems like an odd way to convert a group of people to Christianity.

These strong-arm tactics worked for a while. Many natives stopped drinking kava or used it on the sly when the missionaries weren't around. But by the 1950s the prohibition against kava had pretty much run its course and today kava is no longer viewed as "the devil's drink." In fact, many church officials and island administrators now drink kava regularly with the natives as they have come to realize the benefits of its calming and medicinal properties.

**I'm intrigued. How does kava work? Why does the plant affect the mind and body the way it does?**

The key constituents are kavalactones, also known as kavapyrones. Kavalactones are the active ingredients that give kava its calming effects; they reduce anxiety and improve mood by affecting the brain and body. At least 15 different kavalactones have been isolated, 6 of which—kawain, methysticin, demethoxy-yangonin, dihydrokawain, dihydromethysicin, and yangonin—are known to possess psychoactive effects. According to researchers, all kavalactones can affect the human body, but it is the fat-soluble kavalactones found in kava resin that have the strongest impact on the nervous system. Quality kava roots typically contain between 5 to 8 percent kavalactones.

Researchers still are not sure exactly how kava works, although recent brain tissue studies at the Institute for Physiology and Chemistry at the University of Essen in Germany have provided a clearer understanding of the effects of kava on the brain. These studies have revealed that kavalactones can easily enter the brain and that they bind differently to receptors in various brain regions. Those areas most readily affected by kava include the hippocampus (which is involved in memory and emotions), the amygdala (which responds to emotional stress and alarm), and the medulla oblongata (which helps to regulate body functions such as respiration and circulation). Not surprisingly, kava (unlike other drugs) has little effect on the cerebellum, which is involved in coordination and balance, or the frontal cortex, which affects higher thinking and analytical powers. Other components found in kava also appear to go directly to muscle tissue, which explains the physical relaxation experienced by kava users. These findings help to explain why kava users who consume kava in moderation experience a sense of calm or tranquility but no dizziness, incoordination, or fuzzy thinking.

Researchers at the University of Essen made another startling observation: Kava influences gamma-aminobutyric acid (GABA) receptors in the brain. This finding is important because it may help to explain how kava eases stress and anxiety and promotes sociability. A number of man-made medications also affect GABA receptors. For example, diazepam (Valium)—one of the most popular sedatives in the world—affects GABA receptors, making us feel more relaxed and sleepy. According to German researchers, kava may work in a similar fashion, although additional studies will be needed to confirm this. Other researchers speculate that kava works by interfering with the activity of chemicals such as dopamine, norepinephrine, or serotonin in the brain, which could be instrumental in the herb's ability to reduce anxiety.

## Why have researchers taken so long to analyze kava and its effects on the body? They've known about the herb for 200 years.

Research into kava really isn't a new phenomenon. Scientists were evaluating the various components of kava as long ago as the late 1800s, when methysticin and yangonin were first isolated. It was also around that time that researchers began to notice kava's ability to relax muscles without blocking nerve signals or otherwise affecting the thinking process. Other kavalactones were discovered by German researchers between 1914 and 1933, but it wasn't until 1966 that a German pharmacologist named H. J. Meyer proved that kavalactones were responsible for the plant's psychoactive effects.

Kava research has escalated dramatically in recent years as more and more people worldwide turn to the herb for its social and medicinal benefits (see Chapters 4 and 5 for an in-depth look at studies on kava and stress, anxiety, insomnia, and other medical conditions). Many of the recent clinical studies of kava used a standardized extract known as WS 1490, or Laitan, manufactured by the German drug company Dr. Willmar Schwabe GmbH. The extract contains about 70 milligrams of kavalactones per capsule. This is approximately ten times the amount of kavalactones found in the root—something to keep in mind when shopping for kava.

Consumers should recognize that there can be substantial differences in combinations and levels of ingredients from one kava product to another and that most commercial products will not contain the concentrations of kavalactones used in clinical studies of the plant. According to herbal researchers, many factors can affect the composition of commercial kava products, including the age of the plant upon harvest, the species of kava, the soil and altitude in which it was planted, and the part of the plant used (most companies use ground kava root because it contains the greatest concentrations of kavalactones). We'll discuss these issues again in Chapter 7: Shopping for Kava.

# TWO

❧

## Stress and Anxiety

*FACT:* Stress can dramatically affect your physical health and mental well-being.

*FACT:* People who have trouble dealing with stress become sick four times more often than those with good coping skills.

*FACT:* Health problems related to stress are some of the most common seen by doctors.

*FACT:* An estimated 60 million Americans experience at least some symptoms of anxiety each year, and nearly 30 million Americans have full-blown anxiety disorders.

*FACT:* According to a recent Gallup poll, nearly 25 percent of the American workforce is afflicted with stress and related anxiety—at a cost of $75 billion a year to American businesses.

❧

*Meet Brian. He's 42, an accountant with the same shoe manufacturer that employs our friend Betty from Chapter 1, and a poster boy for the detrimental effects of stress.*

*While Betty had a bad day, Brian has been having a bad month with no letup in sight. There are persistent rumors of impending cutbacks in the accounting department and since Brian was the last to be hired, he's afraid he'll be the first to be fired. Year-end fiscal reports have kept him chained to his desk for the past two weeks, forcing him to skip lunch on most days and work long past quitting time to make sure everything stays on schedule. At home, Brian's wife spends most of the evening nagging him about his long hours at work, his lousy salary, and the fact that they haven't gone on a real vacation in two years. His ten-year-old son is doing poorly in school, and the orthodontist says the boy needs expensive dental work. Then there's the weird noise the car has been making the past few days, a note from Brian's in-laws regarding their plans to drop by for an extended stay, and angry noises from the Internal Revenue Service over last year's tax return.*

*Needless to say, Brian hasn't been feeling well lately. He suffers from persistent insomnia, recurrent indigestion, and floundering libido. He's chronically tired, uncharacteristically irritable, and he always seems to be recovering from a cold or other malady.*

*In short, Brian is yet another victim of hectic twentieth-century living.*

There are good and bad kinds of stress, but most of us experience only the bad kind. In our rush to do our jobs and live our lives, we find ourselves confronted with stressful situations and growing anxiety at almost every turn. Problems in traffic aggravate us on the ride to work in the morning and on the ride home in the evening. Corporate downsizing places additional work and responsibilities on already overburdened employees. Lackadaisical or surly clerks make shopping an irritating chore rather than a pleasure. Add to all of this the ceaseless demands of family and home and it becomes clear why problems associated with stress and anxiety are some of the most common complaints heard by doctors. We're killing ourselves trying to live.

But it doesn't have to be this way. There are proven methods for reducing the stress and anxiety in our lives and making life something to look forward to rather than something to dread. In this chapter, we'll discuss the effects of stress and anxiety on the body, the importance of the mind-body connection, and proven techniques for eliminating stress and anxiety from our lives.

## What is stress?

Unfortunately, the stress that many of us experience is often the result of the full, busy lives that we lead. While not every item in a hectic schedule is necessarily a cause of stress, it is inevitable that balancing so many different demands will impact on our physical, mental, and emotional well-being. Stress can occur suddenly, such as after a near-collision on the freeway, or be more chronic, such as working in a job you hate, dealing daily with a problem child, or trying to cope with an emotional burden such as the death of a loved one or divorce. Stress can also come from environmental factors such as extreme weather, physical illness, or distressing encounters.

The body and mind react to these pressures with what researchers call the "stress response," a phrase coined by Canadian endocrinologist Dr. Hans Selye, who was one of the first to document the various ways the body responds to distressing stimuli. Through his research at McGill University in Montreal, Dr. Selye found that the stress response occurs within the entire body, not just one organ or body part—and that these responses are usually pretty predictable. Typical physiological responses to sudden stress, such as nearly being struck by a bus, include increased heart rate, rapid breathing, muscular tension, sweating, and cold hands or feet. Chronic stress may manifest itself as continual anxiety, physical illness, depression, and mental despair. In extreme situations, chronic stress can even be fatal by worsening serious medical conditions.

## Is all stress bad?

No. Life is full of "good stress," the kind that helps us enjoy certain activities and ultimately grow as individuals and as a species. Dr. Selye called this beneficial form of stress "eustress." A good example of eustress is the thrill you feel when you watch an exciting sporting event such as a close baseball game. Your body experiences a genuine stress response—especially if your team is losing—but it certainly won't hurt you. In fact, if your team wins, you'll feel pretty good!

Participating in an athletic event is even more stressful, but most professional athletes use this sensation of high arousal to psyche themselves up so they will play their best. Entertainers such as actors, singers, and comedians face stress every time they walk out on stage, but the majority say that this stress quickly gives way to a sense of excitement that enhances their performance. Even writers, who live a relatively calm and sedentary lifestyle working at their typewriter or computer, face stress every time they accept an assignment with a deadline. In most cases, however, this kind of low-level stress makes people in artistic occupations even more creative and thus more excited about their work.

Researchers note that many of the most pleasurable things on earth are stressful. Being in love, having passionate sex, working out at the gym—all of these are, strictly speaking, stressful events. The difference is that they make us feel good or are otherwise good for us, both physically and emotionally. We enjoy these activities, so we don't really feel the stressful effects they have on our minds and bodies. As a rule of thumb, if a stressful situation leaves you feeling excited, invigorated, and in good spirits, it's healthy. If it leaves you with a feeling of dread or frustration, it's potentially dangerous and steps should be taken to alleviate it.

## Should we strive for a life completely free of stress? Would that make us more healthy?

It's nearly impossible to live a life completely free of stress, and you probably wouldn't like it anyway because a

100 percent stress-free life would be extremely boring. We would never experience any of the wonderful, exciting, exhilarating things that make life the joy it is. We would simply exist, and that's no way to live. We need at least a little stress in our lives to keep things interesting. It's only when stress levels threaten to get beyond our control that we need to take action.

## You've mentioned a lot of common stressors. Has anyone ever rated the impact of stressful situations faced by the average person?

Actually, yes. In the mid-1960s, two psychiatrists, Thomas Holmes and Richard Rahe, created the Social Readjustment Rating Scale, which measures the severity of change (read: stress) for the average person. Their list contained 43 common life changes and a mean value score for each ranging from 1 to 100. According to Holmes and Rahe, the top ten most stressful life events were death of a spouse (100), divorce (73), marital separation (65), detention in jail or other institution (63), death of a close family member (63), major personal injury or illness (53), marriage (50), being fired from work (47), marital reconciliation (45), and retirement from work (45).

## Can chronic stress make us sick?

Absolutely. Dr. Selye's research found that negative daily stress—the kind experienced by many American workers—can take a heavy toll on the body. Nonstop stress and anxiety wastes energy, places us in a condition of chronic exhaustion, and affects the immune system so that we are at greater risk of illness. A recent Harvard University study confirmed this by noting that people who have trouble coping with stress become sick four times more often than people who handle stress well.

Recurrent colds or other infections are a fairly accurate health indicator that you're experiencing too much stress in your life. Others include daily headaches, incessant worrying, a feeling of constant nervousness, poor concentration, sleep difficulties, irritability or outright anger, constipation or diarrhea, chronic indigestion, and a propensity toward overeating or excessive smoking or drinking.

Of course, unrelenting stress can cause even more serious health problems, including increased risk of heart attack and stroke. Researchers say one reason for this is that a constant flow of adrenalin (epinephrine)—a result of the so-called fight-or-flight mechanism that accompanies a stressful situation—can damage artery walls, thereby promoting the accumulation of fatty deposits. Too much adrenalin can also weaken the heart muscle and increase one's risk of heart attack, even in people with no previous history of heart disease.

If stress continues uncontrolled, the body tries to adapt by adopting a defensive posture for what it perceives as a long-term battle. The pituitary gland (located at the base of the brain) rallies the body's immune forces to fight disease, and various physiologic changes can be noted, including increased blood pressure and arterial constriction and an increase in metabolism and elevated corticosteroid levels, which increase blood platelet levels that in turn can clog arteries. Corticosteroids raise blood sugar levels so we have the energy we need to fight or flee if necessary (a throwback to the days of prehistory when daily survival virtually depended on the fight-or-flight response), but persistent blood sugar spikes can also place us at increased risk for diabetes.

In addition, studies suggest that prolonged negative stress can stimulate the production of free radicals, which are reactive chemicals associated with aging, degenerative disease, and even the formation of certain types of cancer. There is also greater risk of osteoporosis, irritable bowel syndrome, peptic ulcers, and reduced memory and concentration skills. And when you do get sick, it usually takes longer for the body to recover.

The battle against constant negative stress is one the body simply can't win. Eventually a rebound effect sets in, characterized by physical and mental exhaustion, increased vulnerability to illness, and decreased resilience to further stress. Exhaustion is the body's last-ditch effort to tell the mind, "Enough's enough! I need to rest and take care of myself!"

## I'm tired all the time. Could my fatigue be caused by stress in my life?

Very possibly—especially if the stress is constant and unrelenting. The body goes through several phases when faced with continuous stress, and chronic fatigue is an important indicator that you really need to rest and let the body recover.

Not surprisingly, stress-related fatigue is one of the most common health problems facing Americans today. Work, family, and outside activities place a constant demand on our time and physical and mental resources, resulting in a stress response that may not be readily apparent but which affects our health and well-being nonetheless.

## What are some of the most common symptoms of stress-related fatigue or exhaustion?

They are numerous, and many of them mimic symptoms of other ailments. But if you find that you have more than just a few, chances are good that your body is reaching over-load and desperately needs a chance to slow down and repair itself. Some of the most common physical and mental indicators of fatigue include ongoing fear or anxiety, incessant worrying, a general feeling of poor health, bore-dom or low-grade depression, irritability or uncharacteristic bursts of anger or rage, reduced attention span, a decrease in libido, a dependence on alcohol or drugs (both legal and illegal), impaired memory, poor physical condition, reduced stamina, chronic headaches and/or indigestion, and dull complexion.

## Can stress affect sleep patterns as well?

Absolutely. Stress can have a serious impact on our natural body rhythms, resulting in insomnia and other sleep disturbances. People who are under constant pressure, either physically or mentally, may have trouble falling asleep, sleep fitfully, or wake up too early and find themselves unable to fall back to sleep again. As a result, these individuals feel constantly tired during the day, which can have an adverse effect on their ability to perform at work and at home. Simple projects suddenly become extremely difficult, minor irritations become almost overwhelming, and relationships can suffer. People close to exhaustion may feel that nothing they do is good enough, develop a defeatist attitude, or become overly defensive.

We'll discuss the causes and treatment of insomnia and related sleep disorders in greater detail in Chapter 3: Insomnia.

## You mentioned earlier that stress can have a detrimental effect on relationships. How does this happen?

There are a number of ways, though poor communication is one of the most common. Stressed individuals are so overwhelmed by work or other stress-inducing situations that they start neglecting their spouse and loved ones in a desperate attempt to take care of their "problems." People under stress may grow distant, withdraw into themselves, and spend increasing periods away from their families as they struggle to cope. When confronted, they become angry or defensive—perhaps without even realizing it—which distances them even more. The spouse, not really knowing or understanding the cause of their partner's problems, may take the withdrawal as personal rejection and also start putting up walls. Before long, communication becomes all but impossible and the relationship suffers greatly.

A similar dynamic can occur at work as overstressed employees, perhaps focused on the project at hand, unintentionally reject or antagonize coworkers and superiors. They keep to themselves; miss deadlines, are less productive, and blame others for their inability to get the job done. They may also miss a lot of work time due to stress-related illness.

Of course, discussing the causes of stress in your life is one of the best ways to cope with your problems. Keeping the lines of communication open will strengthen your relationships at home and at work. Letting people know you're under a lot of pressure helps them understand your behavior and perhaps offer needed assistance. Very often, the easing of stress is a group endeavor. If you find yourself starting to become overwhelmed, don't hold it in—talk about it. And don't hesitate to ask for help.

## I often hear the word "anxiety" used in discussions about stress. What is anxiety?

Medically speaking, anxiety is an intense state of worry, distress, or apprehension. It is frequently a side effect of daily stress, although mental health officials consider anxiety a predominant symptom in a number of psychiatric conditions with various manifestations and syndromes.

Anxiety disorders range from low-grade anxiety that is produced in adjustment to a transient stressor to more severe conditions such as panic disorder, agoraphobia (an irrational fear of being in public places), post-traumatic stress disorder, specific phobias, social phobia, obsessive-compulsive disorder, or generalized anxiety disorder. Health officials say these conditions produce some of the most common medical complaints in the United States, and antianxiety medications have been among the most frequently prescribed medications in the United States for several decades. As our society and culture becomes increasingly stressful, the number of people with related anxiety problems escalates. It is estimated that more than 60 million Americans experience at least some symptoms of anxiety each year, and nearly 30 million have a fully-realized clinical anxiety disorder.

When discussing anxiety in this book, we will be referring primarily to generalized anxiety, with symptoms that afflict most of us at some time in our lives.

## What are the most common symptoms of anxiety?

Common psychological symptoms of generalized anxiety include feelings of alarm, dread, fear, worry, anger, and panic. Physical symptoms include accelerated heart rate at rest, trembling, restlessness, sweaty hands, stomach distress, diarrhea, headache, rapid breathing, faintness, dizziness, and a numbness or tingling sensation in the hands or feet.

It's important to note that anxiety comes in many forms and varies in type and severity of symptoms. It can strike when least expected (often leading to a panic attack), or it can be a constant companion, ever present like your shadow.

## Is anxiety always bad?

There are two kinds of anxiety: the normal kind everyone experiences when confronting a challenge or facing the unknown, and chronic, persistent anxiety, which is never healthy and can lead to illness.

Everyone experiences occasional anxiety; it's just a part of living. And very often stress and anxiety go hand in hand. Students facing a test, for example, may experience fear, panic, sweaty hands, and an upset stomach—especially if they haven't studied! Entertainers who perform before a live audience may have similar symptoms; some become so anxious that they feel nauseous or throw up before walking on stage. An employee whose job is in jeopardy will likely also experience symptoms of anxiety, as will someone going through a major life crisis, such as a serious illness, the death of a loved one, or relationship problems. In cases such as these, the symptoms of anxiety are generally self-limited and usually disappear once the issue has been resolved.

Chronic anxiety may be low-grade and evident only under stress or duress, or it may be omnipresent and nearly incapacitating. Regardless of degree, chronic anxiety can have a detrimental effect on nearly every aspect of our lives. It can make us ill, prevent us from getting needed rest and affect our work and important relationships. Very often, nothing short of medication or therapy can alleviate it.

## How does anxiety affect the body?

Anxiety, like stress, can affect almost every system in the human body, although, as with almost anything, people react to it differently. Some experience only minor symptoms, while others are plagued with anxiety-related health problems so severe that they interfere with daily living.

Anxiety can cause our heart rate to fluctuate wildly and our blood pressure to rise. It can interfere with digestion (people with anxiety are often afflicted with constipation or diarrhea) and trigger sudden and prolonged headaches. It can cause significant muscle tension. It can dramatically affect the sex drive and cause significant sleep disturbances, including insomnia. It can make us eat too much, or suddenly lose weight. In short, anxiety can be an "all over" problem, and that can make an accurate diagnosis difficult.

## Who suffers from anxiety problems more often— men or women?

According to national health officials, more than twice as many women are afflicted with anxiety problems as men, although the reason for this difference is unknown. It could be that women are simply more prone to anxious feelings, or that men just don't admit to them as often as women. However, studies show that men are more likely than women to cope with anxiety through the use of alcohol and drugs. As an aside, it should be noted that anxiety takes a heavy toll on American businesses. A recent Gallup poll revealed that nearly 25 percent of the workforce is afflicted with anxiety and related stress—at a cost of $75 billion a year.

## Do most people with anxiety get the help they need?

Sadly, no. Anxiety is often very easy to treat through medication, therapy, or alternative approaches such as herbalism, but many people suffering from anxiety go their entire lives without seeking help. In many cases, people with anxiety refrain from seeing a doctor because they're afraid of being labeled insane, or they're convinced they can keep their problem under control by themselves. Of course, people who suffer from generalized anxiety aren't insane, but the fear of being labeled as such is a strong deterrent. And self-treating anxiety by holding it in or assuming it will go away on its own seldom works; usually, this approach only results in additional health problems.

Anxiety is a common ailment, is nothing to be ashamed of, and is very treatable. If you suffer from symptoms that indicate an anxiety disorder, see a doctor at once.

## I worry a lot. Does this mean I have an anxiety disorder?

Maybe, maybe not. It depends on the degree to which your worrying affects your life and whether or not it is accompanied by physical symptoms of anxiety. In other words, is worrying something you do only occasionally and for justifiable reasons, or is it persistent, usually over trivial matters, and almost impossible to control?

Everyone worries about problems in their life; that's completely natural. We worry about our children's safety when they're away from us, and we worry about whether or not we'll get that raise we've worked so hard for. Worrying is both a way of solving problems (by thinking hard about a problem, we often can come up with the answer) and of coping with situations that very often we can do nothing about.

Chronic, inescapable worrying, especially about issues that can't be helped or wouldn't trouble others in similar circumstances, could indicate an anxiety disorder. If worry and anxiety are taking over your life, you should definitely consult your doctor. Why suffer when you don't have to?

## Do researchers know what causes anxiety?

They're getting closer and closer every day. One explanation, supported by recent studies, is that anxiety is caused by biochemical overstimulation of the region of the brain known as the amygdala, coupled with fearful thinking. This combination, researchers speculate, leads to an overactive stress response and the physical symptoms most commonly associated with anxiety disorders. This cycle could be a clear example of the mind-body connection: Worrisome thoughts lead to physical symptoms, which in turn fuel more worrisome thoughts. The most successful treatment, say psychiatrists, is a combination of medication therapy and psychotherapy. The medications help to modulate the biochemical problems in the brain, and the therapy both eases and promotes understanding of the worrisome thoughts.

## Could you explain the concept of the mind-body connection and how it applies to stress and anxiety?

Scientific studies have proved again and again that the mind wields amazing control over the body. Just look at the effects of biofeedback. Using a biofeedback machine as a gauge you can, with practice, slow your heart rate, ease pain, and control other bodily functions merely by thinking about it. By the same principle, we can think ourselves sick and we can think ourselves well. Researchers call this the mind-body connection, and an ever-increasing body of evidence suggests it can play a very important role in the development or cure of a wide variety of medical problems, including stress and anxiety.

Not surprisingly, the key to all of this is our emotions. Anger, hostility, sadness, and depression all work to suppress our immune systems and open the door to illness. Happiness, confidence, family support, and an overall positive outlook, on the other hand, can stimulate the immune response and help us overcome disease and other physical problems.

Thinking and worrying about the stress in our lives can easily trigger a stress response with all of the typical physical manifestations, such as headache, stomachache, sweaty palms, and tingly nervousness. It works the same way with anxiety, too. So strong is the mind-body connection that often we can bring on an anxiety attack simply by thinking about a situation that makes us anxious. And the more we think about it, the more anxious we become.

But as we now know, the mind-body connection can also act as a healer. People with chronic anxiety problems should see a doctor, but those who suffer only occasionally from anxiety may find that they can ward off an impending attack simply by thinking themselves calm. A relaxing walk, a hot bath, a soothing massage, passionate sex, and meditation in a quiet, serene environment are all excellent ways to stop anxiety or stress from taking control. The key is to think pleasant, happy, nonstressful thoughts until both your mind and body are uniformly calm. It takes practice, but it really does work.

### My father is extremely anxious, and as I grow older I find myself following in his shoes. Can anxiety be hereditary?

A growing number of clinical studies suggest that a predisposition to anxiety may be hereditary. In fact, the risk of panic attacks—a feature of one type of anxiety disorder— has been shown to be about eight times higher among familial relations than in the general public, which suggests a strong genetic connection. In unrelated studies, researchers have found that nearly 40 percent of people afflicted with agoraphobia have a close relative with some sort of anxiety disorder, and if one identical twin has panic disorder, there's a 40 percent chance the other twin will have it too.

Indeed, a genetic predisposition to anxiety makes sense. After all, researchers have identified genes that appear to contribute to neuroticism and obsessive-compulsive disorder, so why not generalized anxiety? But it must be noted that having the gene for a particular anxiety problem does not necessarily mean a person will develop the disorder. Researchers say environment, physical factors, and personality also play an important role in determining whether or not an anxiety problem will arise.

**I suffer from occasional bouts of generalized anxiety, which I control with medication. Over the years I've found that whenever I'm around someone who is sad or angry, I tend to assume those negative emotions. Is this common?**

More common than you might imagine. Studies have found that people afflicted with anxiety are very susceptible to the negative emotions of others and that they can, if they're not careful, assume those emotions. The next time you find yourself feeling bad or overwhelmed by negative feelings, check those around you. Are they angry at life? Chronic complainers? Always unhappy? If so, try to separate yourself from that environment. If that is not possible, mentally disassociate yourself from such emotions by thinking about things in life that make you happy or joyful until the negative feelings disappear.

**Since anxiety is so common in the general public, are most doctors pretty adept at diagnosing and treating it?**

Unfortunately, the answer is no. Several studies have found that the majority of anxious people who finally do seek help for their physical symptoms visit several doctors in various specialties before their problem is accurately diagnosed and treated. There are several reasons for this. First, the symptoms of anxiety are very frequently seen in other disorders, and if someone specializes in a particular area, say gastroenterology, they typically look for problems in their specialty before branching out. In addition, because of our current system of managed care, many doctors outside of psychiatry are simply too busy to properly evaluate, diagnose, and treat someone with an anxiety disorder.

If you believe you have an anxiety problem and are seeking treatment, you can help yourself by answering your doctor's evaluation form as thoroughly and accurately as possible. Tell your doctor everything you can about your symptoms and concerns (lying or avoiding the issue helps no one), and don't forget to mention any drugs or supplements that you may be taking. This includes prescription and over-the-counter medications, herbs, and also illegal drugs. Your doctor should also give you a thorough physical exam to rule out any medical cause for your condition.

## How is generalized anxiety typically diagnosed?

Like most health problems with no clear cause, doctors confirm generalized anxiety through what is known as a differential diagnosis, in which all potential causes, both physical and mental, are gradually eliminated until generalized anxiety disorder remains the most likely culprit. Anxiety is a symptom of nearly all psychiatric conditions, but the more serious problems, such as schizophrenia or panic disorder, have other identifying features that set them apart.

## Is anxiety always a psychiatric illness? Can it also be caused by any specific diseases or health problems?

Actually, a number of physical maladies can trigger or closely mimic anxiety symptoms. For example, mitral valve prolapse, a relatively common and usually harmless irregularity in a heart valve, can place someone at greater risk of panic attacks. Anxiety can also be caused by pain associated with coronary disease and angina pectoris, abnormal heart rhythms, and other cardiac disorders; hyperthyroidism; hypoglycemia; emphysema, pulmonary edema, pulmonary thrombosis, asthma, or other respiratory disorders; menopause; and vertigo.

A large number of drugs have also been associated with anxiety including alcohol, amphetamines, caffeine, cocaine, antihistamines, antihypertensives, dopamine, ephedrine, methylphenidate, salicylates, glucocorticoids, thyroid agents, and others, as well as the herb yohimbine. If you are on a medication and suddenly experience anxiety symptoms, see your doctor immediately. If it's the medication that's causing your problems, a less reactive substitute can usually be found.

## Is there a correlation between anxiety and depression?

Yes, a very strong one. Mental health officials note that chronically anxious people often plunge into a deep depression because they can't seem to cope with life situations that others handle with seemingly no trouble at all.

Anxiety and depression—which share a number of common symptoms—often work as a team to ruin a person's life. Anxious people become depressed over the symptoms of their disorder, and the depression may make them even more anxious. A depressed individual can also develop secondary anxiety. That's why it's so important that someone afflicted with anxiety get help as soon as possible.

Studies show that people with certain types of anxiety disorders are more prone to depressive episodes than others. Agoraphobics—people who become nervous or anxious at the thought of going out in public—are especially prone to depression. So are people afflicted with panic disorder; nearly half of people who have multiple attacks eventually develop a serious bout of depression. Depression is also commonly seen in individuals with post-traumatic stress disorder, obsessive-compulsive disorder, and social phobia.

Doctors believe that low levels of the brain hormone serotonin play an important role in both disorders in some people. Thankfully, there are number of drugs—known as selective serotonin reuptake inhibitors (SSRIs)—that can help. The most commonly prescribed medications in this class include fluoxetine (Prozac), paroxetine (Paxil), sertra-line (Zoloft), and fluvoxamine (Luvox). St. John's Wort, an herb that has developed an international reputation as a mild antidepressant, may also be effective in certain individuals afflicted with both anxiety and depression.

**Could you please provide more information on some of the other anxiety-related problems mentioned in this chapter, such as panic disorder and phobias?**

The disorders you mention are two of the more common and distressing anxiety conditions seen by doctors and usu-ally require treatment with medication, psychotherapy, and/or other interventions. Kava and other alternative ther-apies may be somewhat helpful, but in more severe cases medical and psychiatric intervention remains the key to successful treatment.

Panic disorder is characterized by a sudden and often overwhelming feeling of terror and apprehension accompa-nied by physical symptoms throughout the body such as a racing heart and palpitations, shortness of breath, dizziness and lightheadedness, sweaty palms, headache, and nausea. This is anxiety in one of its severest forms, and it can be ter-rifying and, at times, incapacitating.

Typically, panic attacks begin without warning and are often triggered by a seemingly nonstressful activity outside the home such as driving a car, entering a store, or working at one's desk. The victims feel lightheaded and sweaty and are overcome by feelings of terror and impending doom. They may feel like they are smothering or choking, and they may experience a painful tightening in the chest that's frighteningly similar to a heart attack. Many panic attack patients say they actually feel like they are dying and that there is nothing they can do to control it. Most panic attacks last less than ten minutes, and the majority of peo-ple recover fully within a half-hour. In a great many cases, fatigue sets in following an intense panic attack.

Approximately 1 to 2 percent of the population experience recurring panic attacks, with onset typically occurring in the late teens and early 20s. As mentioned earlier, panic disorder has a familial risk. If someone is diagnosed with panic disorder, up to 18 percent of first-degree relatives are likely to have the condition, too. Twins are especially susceptible.

Severe panic attacks can take a heavy toll on someone's life, especially if they occur with frequency. Some people develop what is known as anticipatory anxiety and strive to avoid those situations that have been associated with panic attacks in the past. And many people—especially women by a two to one ratio to men—develop agoraphobia, defined as an irrational fear of being alone or in public places. Needless to say, this combination can have an extreme effect on work and family relations. Other potential complications include depression and substance abuse.

Phobias are divided into two general classes: simple phobias and social phobias. Simple phobias are persistent irrational fears and avoidance of specific objects or situations, such as a fear of heights, closed spaces, or flying. In general, these are a common problem—a lot of people dislike snakes, bugs, or high places—and diagnosis of a true phobic disorder is usually made only when the phobia has a significant impact on a person's life. Gradual exposure and desensitization is the most effective treatment for simple phobias, which usually don't respond to medication. When fear of an object, place, or situation prevents you from enjoying life, it's probably time to see a doctor.

Social phobia is characterized by an irrational fear and avoidance of situations in which a person may be potentially judged, embarrassed, criticized, or humiliated in front of others, such as a fear of public speaking or an inability to urinate in a public restroom (a problem commonly known as shy bladder syndrome). For many victims of social phobia even the possibility of such a situation can trigger terrifying anxiety that dramatically impacts on a person's lifestyle. Luckily, most people with social phobia react well to therapy with gradual desensitization. There is also a mounting body of evidence supporting the use of medication to treat social phobia.

## My job has really been getting to me lately, and I'm afraid the stress is going to make me sick. Can you suggest some effective coping techniques?

There are a number of simple and effective ways to cope with daily stress and prevent it from making you ill. Foremost, you must recognize the sources of stress in your life and do what you can to eliminate or at least reduce them. If your job is a pressure cooker and you find yourself dreading going to the office every day, perhaps it's time to find a less stressful job. Many people stay in jobs they loathe because they are making good money, but in the long run they pay a terrible price as stress destroys their health and wrecks their most cherished personal relationships.

If it's those same personal relationships that are the source of your stress, do what you must to fix them. Discuss your problems and possible solutions in a neutral, non-threatening place (a restaurant, for example), and don't hesitate to seek counseling if you think it will help. Most family and relationship problems can be remedied through effective communication and sincere negotiation.

For most people, though, daily stress is really an accumulation of small, niggling problems—a broken shoelace, car problems, a sick child, a fast-approaching deadline at work, a malfunctioning air conditioner at home. By themselves, none of these is a serious problem. But taken as a whole, they can trigger a major stress response.

There are a lot of ways to cope with the small problems we face in everyday life. The first—and most effective—is to consciously refuse to let them bother you. Address each problem as it comes and fix it as best as you can before addressing the next. Letting problems accumulate with the intention of taking care of them later only leads to more stress. Make "I will not let stress dominate my life" become your personal daily mantra.

It's also a good idea to schedule a little relaxation time for yourself every day. Too often we work all day, come home and work long into the night, fall into bed, wake up, and begin the cycle again. We don't give ourselves time to relax and calm down. So pick a time each day and make it yours. It could be first thing in the morning before you go to work, an hour before or after dinner, or immediately before you go to bed. Always remember—this is *your* time. Take a relaxing bath, listen to calming music, catch up on your recreational reading, have your mate give you a back rub (or use your time together for a little relaxing intimacy), or meditate. The key is to reduce external stress and stimulation so that your body has a chance to slow down and recharge. Practice this daily and before you know it, you will have eliminated a great deal of negative stress, and you'll be ready to face each day with a renewed love of life.

The following are some simple changes in lifestyle that can also help you cope with stress. They may seem like commonsense tips, but you'd be surprised at how many people don't follow them.

- **Eat a balanced diet.** Fatty foods, sugar, caffeine, and alcohol only enhance the physical effects of stress; try to cut down or eliminate them altogether. Instead, fill your plate with lots of poultry, fresh fruits and vegetables, and pasta. You'll be amazed at the impact your diet has on your physical and mental well-being.

- **Stop smoking.** Nicotine is a stimulant that no one needs. It's also harmful to your heart and lungs.

- **Get plenty of sleep.** Easier said than done when your life is full of stress, but there are ways to make it happen. We'll discuss them in greater detail in Chapter 3: Insomnia.

- **Get sufficient exercise.** Stressed people often say they just don't have the time to exercise, but you must *make* the time. And you don't have to join a gym or buy a lot of expensive exercise equipment to become more physically active. A brisk walk around the block can be an invigorating experience. Other options include swimming, bicycling, tennis, and aerobics. An hour or so three times a week is adequate, but the more you exercise the better you'll feel because exercise is a wonderful stress buster. It tones your heart and muscles, stimulates the production of mood-altering brain chemicals called endorphins, and promotes sound sleep.

- **Take steps to avoid stressful situations and individuals.** If the drive to work is killing you, take public transportation or join a car pool. If a coworker is driving you nuts, see if you can move your desk. Remember, you don't have to take it. For almost every stressful situation, there's a calming alternative.

- **Spend a few minutes each day at work engaging in some stress-reducing guided imagery.** Shut your office door, turn down the lights, close your eyes, and mentally place yourself in a quiet, serene, and enjoyable location, such as a Caribbean beach or a mountain cabin—any place where stress can't find you.

- **Take a vacation.** Get away from all the sources of your daily stress and enjoy yourself. Don't take work with you and don't tell your boss where you'll be staying—otherwise, what's the point in getting away? Instead, bring that book you've been dying to read, find a comfortable cabana on a quiet beach (or any other soothing location), and let the stress melt from your mind and body. The Europeans understand the value of vacations in the workplace and most workers get several weeks of vacation time each year. Americans can learn a lot from that kind of thinking. In addition to extended vacations, make it a habit to get away for a fun weekend occasionally with your spouse, even if it's just to a hotel across town. A change of scenery, even for only a couple of days, can have a tremendous impact on our physical and emotional health.

**I have a problem with anxiety. It doesn't strike often and isn't serious enough to require medication, but it can be a hassle when it comes over me. Could you offer some tips on how to deal with low-grade anxiety?**

Let me begin by reiterating the fact that everyone experiences some degree of anxiety in their daily lives—it's an inescapable part of contemporary living, and most people deal with it quite easily. In fact, a little anxiety can be a good thing in that it often helps us make important decisions. But when anxiety adversely affects behavior, mental and emotional judgment and enjoyment of life, it's time to consult a doctor.

There are many effective ways to deal with the most common kind of anxiety, that general feeling of apprehension or worry that afflicts us at work and at home. As with stress, the most important thing is to recognize that you are anxious and try to determine the cause. Is your boss putting more pressure on you to produce at work? Are you, your spouse, or your child ill? Are you experiencing financial problems? Uncovering the source of your anxiety is the first step in making it better. If external factors are the cause, your anxiety should disappear once those problems are corrected. This is especially true of anxiety caused by environmental factors, but also of physical illness or certain medications, as discussed earlier.

A lot of anxiety is caused by guilt. If you're experiencing low-grade, generalized anxiety for no apparent reason, ask yourself if you've wronged someone at work or at home. If the answer is yes, do what you must to make amends. A clear conscience fosters little anxiety.

Many of the coping mechanisms discussed above for stress are also applicable for low-grade, generalized anxiety. A more healthful diet, increased exercise, satisfactory sleep, and a reduction in tobacco and alcohol consumption can all ease feelings of anxiety by boosting mood-altering chemicals in the brain and improving your general health. Of course, if your anxiety is caused by overwhelming stress in your life—a common problem in contemporary society—then eliminating those stressors should also have a positive effect on feelings of anxiety.

## Is therapy with medication an effective means of controlling stress and anxiety? What are the most common medications prescribed for these problems?

Medications can be very effective in treating persistent anxiety and related stress, although in cases of clinical generalized anxiety disorder, doctors are encouraged to first try nonpharmacological approaches to treatment, such as supportive or cognitive-behavioral psychotherapy.

Barbiturates, a family of very strong sedative/hypnotics, were the drug of choice for the treatment of anxiety until the mid-1950s. They were problematic—users risked a long list of potential side effects including oversedation, overdose, and addiction—but barbiturates were pretty much all that was available until researchers developed more user-friendly medications such as diazepam (Valium), a benzodiazepine sedative that quickly became one of the most widely prescribed medications in the United States, especially among women. As proof of the wide popularity of benzodiazepines, consider that 462,000 pounds of the drugs were consumed in 1958 and a stunning 1.5 million pounds in 1959. Women who were not fulfilled in their at-home role while their husbands were out in the world working were the most frequent users.

Benzodiazepines, which are still in wide use today, were considered safer than heavily-sedating barbiturates, but they were far from perfect. Dependence and addiction remained a problem, and throughout the late 1950s and 1960s, a growing number of people, predominantly women, found themselves hooked on what the Rolling Stones called "mother's little helper." Doctors today are a bit more cautious when it comes to distributing sedatives and hypnotics, but these compounds continue to play an important role in the control of stress and anxiety disorders.

Indeed, when it is determined that generalized anxiety is severe enough to warrant therapy with medication, benzodiazepines remain the most commonly used medications. In many cases, a short course of anxiolytics (anxiety-reducing drugs)—five to seven days—may be all that is necessary to ease overwhelming feelings of anxiety and help the person deal with whatever problems were causing the anxious state. All too frequently, however, these drugs are used for extended periods beyond that needed for the initial anxiety indication and may lead to medication tolerance and dependence. The most commonly used benzodiazepines include chlordiazepoxide (Librium), clonazepam (Klonopin), diazepam (Valium), lorazepam (Ativan), oxazepam (Serax), and alprazolam (Xanax). Shorter-acting benzodiazepines, such as flurazepam (Dalmane), temazepam (Restoril), and triazolam (Halcion), are often used as effective hypnotics or sleep aids.

Newer medications with anxiolytic properties include the following:

- **Beta-adrenergic blocking agents such as propranolol.** Originally developed to treat high blood pressure, these compounds are also used to treat social anxiety and have been found to be especially effective in controlling physical manifestations of anxiety, such as tremors and heart palpitations. However, these drugs are less effective in easing psychological manifestations of anxiety such as intense fearfulness.

- **Azapirones, a new class of anxiolytic drugs that work on the serotoninergic neurotransmitter system.** One of the first in this family was buspirone (Buspar), which appears to ease anxiety symptoms through interaction with serotonin receptors in the brain. Although their onset of action may take several days to weeks to take full effect, azapirones result in far fewer serious side effects (such as sedation, psychomotor impairment, and dependence) than the benzodiazepines.

- **Antidepressants.** While antidepressants are the treatment of choice for several anxiety disorders, their specific role in the treatment of generalized anxiety remains unclear. Medications that have shown some initial promise in this area include imipramine (Tofranil), trazodone (Desyrel), nefazodone (Serzone), paroxetine (Paxil), and venlafaxine (Effexor). These medications remain under investigation for their efficacy in the treatment of generalized anxiety and have not yet received FDA approval for this use.

## What are the most common side effects of the benzodiazepine anxiolytics?

Side effects are relatively rare with benzodiazepines if they are prescribed in low doses and for short periods of time. However, the most commonly reported side effects include muscle incoordination, drowsiness, dizziness, confusion, mild disturbances in perception, and decreased sex drive. In addition, benzodiazepines interact with alcohol, worsening the feelings of intoxication, and in rare cases with overdose, can be fatal.

## I'm pregnant and feeling kind of anxious. Is it okay for me to take a low-dose sedative?

No. Pregnant or breast-feeding women should avoid the use of sedatives because the drugs can affect their fetus or newborn child. Consult your doctor for safer alternatives.

**I've been taking antianxiety medication for awhile, and I feel fine now. Can I just stop taking it?**

Absolutely not. It's essential that you be gradually weaned off of antianxiety medication so as not to go into withdrawal. It isn't fun; symptoms can include nervousness, insomnia, and even seizures. If you wish to discontinue your medication, do so with the assistance of your doctor.

# THREE

―❦―

## *Insomnia*

*FACT:*    Insomnia is one of the most common medical complaints heard by doctors.

*FACT:*    Women experience sleep problems much more often than men, due in part to physiological changes as a result of menstruation, pregnancy, childbirth, breast-feeding, and menopause.

*FACT:*    A prolonged lack of sleep can have a devastating effect on physical and mental well-being.

*FACT:*    It is estimated that one in four American adults and one in two seniors experience occasional or recurrent sleep problems, and those figures will continue to rise as the baby boom generation reaches old age.

*FACT:*    The National Commission on Sleep Disorders estimates that nearly $16 billion is spent annually on problems directly linked to sleep disturbances—and this doesn't include the cost of accidents caused by the people who have become walking zombies as a result of chronic sleep deprivation.

―❦―

*Gretchen can't remember the last time she had a really good night's sleep. Ever since graduating from college and entering the workforce, the 26-year-old assistant bank manager has had trouble falling asleep at night—and sleeping well until morning. On the average evening, Gretchen's mind races for hours, unable to shut down at the end of the day. And when she finally does fall asleep, usually around 1 or 2 AM, she dozes fitfully and awakens frequently. When the alarm clock heralds a new morning at the ungodly hour of 6 AM, Gretchen stumbles out of bed feeling as if she hasn't slept at all. Her mind is a thick fog, her body a mass of aches and pains, and it takes all the willpower she can muster just to shower, get dressed, and get out the door.*

*Gretchen forces a facade of cheerful perkiness when she arrives at the bank promptly at 8 AM. She greets everyone with a smile and a nod, but it's all an act. She'd give anything for the opportunity to climb back into bed and reclaim the sleep that's been denied her for so long. It isn't until after 10 AM and three or four cups of black coffee that Gretchen starts to feel normal again. But even with such a heavy dose of caffeine coursing through it, her body demands a nap around 4 PM every day. By the time Gretchen gets home at 5:30, she's so exhausted she can barely make dinner. Such is her routine every weekday—and most weekends.*

Gretchen suffers from insomnia, which is commonly defined as the inability to fall asleep or stay asleep throughout the night. Almost everyone suffers from sleep problems some time in their lives, but for a growing number of Americans—young and old alike—insomnia is a nightmare so frequent that it routinely affects their mental and physical health.

Indeed, the effects of poor sleep can be many and often quite serious. Lack of sleep places unwanted stress and strain on a number of important organs and body systems, and it weakens our immune response so that we are at greater risk of contracting an infection. Mentally, prolonged sleep deprivation can disrupt the thinking process, dull concentration, and affect memory. Simple tasks become increasingly difficult, and we slowly lose the ability to cope successfully with the everyday stresses of life. Constantly on the verge of exhaustion, we become irritable and testy with loved ones and coworkers until relationships falter and friendships disintegrate.

But insomnia doesn't have to be a lifelong problem. There are numerous ways to reestablish healthy sleep patterns and banish insomnia forever. In this chapter, we'll discuss the many faces of insomnia and related sleep disturbances, the sleep-health connection, and how to overcome insomnia's vicious cycle.

## What is insomnia?

Insomnia is typically defined as the inability to fall asleep or sleep well throughout the night. It may represent a primary sleep disturbance, or it may be secondary to other medical or mental conditions, or to medication use or alcohol or other drug use. Most insomnia is temporary, affecting sleep for a few days to a week or so, then disappearing as suddenly as it arrived. People commonly experience transient insomnia before a big business meeting or on the eve of a new job. Chronic insomnia, which usually lasts several weeks or even months, may occur as a result of more serious life changes such as the birth of a child, divorce, or the death of a loved one. Transient insomnia is rarely dangerous, but chronic insomnia can pose serious health hazards if not treated.

## How common is insomnia?

Extremely common, and growing more so by the year, according to national health officials. Figures vary, but it is estimated that one in four American adults and one in two seniors experience occasional or recurrent sleep problems, and those figures will continue to rise as the baby boom generation reaches old age. Women tend to have more sleep problems than men, due in part to the effects of physiological changes associated with menstruation, pregnancy, childbirth, breast-feeding, and menopause. Not surprisingly, sleep complaints are some of the most common seen by doctors. One dominant factor appears to be our hectic lifestyle—as our lives fill with more and more stress, our ability to get a good night's sleep becomes increasingly difficult.

Sleep disorders have a huge impact on the American and global economy. The National Commission on Sleep Disorders estimates that nearly $16 billion a year is spent on problems directly linked to sleep disorders, and this doesn't include the cost of accidents caused by people whose mental abilities have become grossly impaired as a result of chronic sleep deprivation.

## Before we get into the causes and treatments of insomnia, could you explain the states of sleep and their role in health?

Sleep comes in distinct and definable states and stages, which can be accurately monitored by devices such as the electroencephalogram (EEG), which measures electrical activity in the brain, and the electrooculogram, which measures eye-movement activity.

There are two main states of sleep: non-rapid-eye-movement (NREM) sleep, which has four specific stages, and rapid-eye-movement (REM) sleep. It is typically during REM sleep that we dream most vividly, with our eyes darting wildly back and forth as the mini-movie in our brain plays out. We pass back and forth between these states throughout the night, although the frequency and duration of each is dependent on a number of factors including age, health, medication use, and prior sleep deprivation.

Stage 1 sleep is the light sleep experienced just as we doze off. Sleep is easily interrupted during this stage and we often experience an odd mixture of sleep and wakefulness before falling into deeper sleep. Stage 2 sleep quickly follows, and this is considered the first period of real sleep. After a brief "rest" in stage 2, we fall deeper into stages 3 and 4—known medically as "slow wave sleep" or "delta sleep." Studies suggest that our immune system is most active during these stages, attacking invading bacteria and promoting healing throughout the body. A deficiency in slow wave sleep is often found in seniors, people afflicted with chronic pain, some sleeping pill users, and people with other conditions. Because they are never well-rested, these individuals often have a weakened immune response and are easy prey for infection and other diseases.

Most people achieve stage 4—the deepest level of sleep—about 30 to 45 minutes after falling asleep. We stay in this stage for a short while and then begin our first cycle of REM sleep, during which we have our most abstract and surreal dreams. After a short while, we return to stage 1 to plummet once again into the deeper stages of sleep, starting the process all over again. Most sleep researchers believe that you need at least four uninterrupted sleep cycles consisting of both NREM and REM sleep to awaken feeling fully rested and refreshed.

Interestingly, sleep studies have found that most people spend more time in deep, restful sleep during the first half of the night than in the second half. This is simply the body's way of making sure we get enough priority sleep so that we feel rested and alert in the morning.

## Why do we need sleep, and what happens to our bodies while we're asleep?

Researchers are unsure exactly why we sleep, although we do know it's essential to our survival. A prolonged lack of sleep can have a devastating effect on our physical and mental health and, in extreme cases, can even result in death.

One of the most important purposes of sleep is to let our bodies refuel and regenerate. Many of our body's functions—body temperature, heart rate, blood pressure, digestion—slow dramatically during sleep. But while it may appear that our entire body is completely inactive, the truth is that quite a bit is going on physiologically. The slowing of various systems allows the body's cells to repair, regenerate, and fight disease. In fact, missing just one night of sleep can have a measurable effect on our immune system. In one revealing study, Dr. Michael Irwin of the San Diego Veterans Affairs Medical Center gathered 23 healthy men ages 22 to 61 in a sleep laboratory and let them sleep normally for the first two nights. On the third night, the subjects were kept awake from 3 AM to 7 AM, which is when most of us get our most restful sleep. Dr. Irwin found that the activity of the cells that commonly fight viral infections fell measurably in 18 of the men the morning after they were deprived of sound sleep, proving the importance of sleep in helping to ward off disease. However, the body is a resilient machine, and the effectiveness of the so-called "killer cells" was restored to normal when the subjects were allowed to sleep through the next night without interruption. If just one night of interrupted sleep can have such a strong impact on our immune system, imagine the impact of weeks of poor sleep. That's why people suffering from chronic insomnia seem to get sick all the time.

### Does everyone require the same amount of sleep?

No. Duration and quality of sleep vary dramatically among individuals. Seniors and infants have the most frequent interruptions of sleep, although middle-age adults who are ill or under a lot of stress may also often find their sleep interrupted.

Most healthy adults sleep an average of seven to eight hours a night, although some people get along fine on a little more or a little less. However, too little or too much sleep appears to have a detrimental effect on mortality, doctors note. Studies show that people who sleep fewer than four hours or more than nine hours per night on average have increased mortality rates compared to those who sleep seven to eight hours.

## Do we get the same quality of sleep when we take naps as when we sleep during the night?

Yes, but it depends on how long you snooze. A short nap usually leaves you feeling better than a long one.

Sleep researchers have found that nap sleep is quite similar to nighttime sleep, but because naps tend to be considerably shorter, we don't have enough time to cycle through all the sleep stages. The average 30-minute nap may take us no further than stage 2 sleep. When we awaken, we'll probably feel pretty good—alert, refreshed, and happy. However, if we nap long enough to fall into stage 3 sleep but don't find our way back to stage 1 again, we may awaken feeling lethargic and not particularly well-rested.

## I visited my doctor recently to discuss my occasional insomnia and the terms circadian rhythms, or cycles, kept coming up. I'm not familiar with these terms, and I was too embarrassed to ask for an explanation. What are circadian rhythms, and what is their influence on sleep?

Circadian rhythm is the day-and-night cycle that controls the biological functions of almost all living creatures, both plant and animal. The typical circadian cycle is around 24 hours in length, or the duration of a single day, and it affects dozens of smaller, interrelated cycles within our bodies that keep us in sync with the world around us. In other words, it's the circadian cycle that keeps us awake and active during the day and that lets us fall into sleep at night. Internal rhythms affected by the circadian cycle include hunger, mood, body temperature, immune response, hormone production, and energy levels. Our sleep patterns are also partially controlled by these closely linked internal rhythms. As a result, sudden changes in our internal rhythms, such as from illness or seasonal changes in daylight, can have a noticeable effect on our physical and mental well-being.

Our sleep/wake cycles are controlled by two important glands in the brain—the pineal gland and the hypothalamus. The pineal gland senses when day gives way to night and releases chemicals to help us sleep, such as melatonin. As a result of these hormonal chemicals, our body temperatures drop, our heart rate slows, we feel fatigued and, if everything goes as planned, we slowly fall into a deep and restful sleep. As the first rays of daylight enter our bedroom, the pineal gland stops the production of melatonin so that we wake up. The hypothalamus is signaled to the presence of light through the retinas in our eyes, and this signal is transmitted to the pineal gland. As a result, the pineal gland's ability to sense changes in light and dark plays an integral role in our circadian cycle. People who are blind often have sleep problems associated with their brains' inability to detect these differences.

The influence of the circadian rhythm on our lives, as you might imagine, is profound. Researchers have had volunteers spend extended periods in a cave with no clocks and have found that when people don't have outside light as a gauge, they lose track of time and develop longer sleep/wake patterns—sometimes as long as 33 hours. However, their internal clocks often continue to run on a traditional 24-hour cycle, resulting in problems ranging from lethargy to feelings of disorientation or confusion.

## What kinds of sleep problems can result when circadian rhythms are disrupted?

There are many, say sleep researchers. One disorder, called delay sleep phase syndrome, results from a slower than normal circadian rhythm and is characterized by the inability to fall asleep at the proper time. In extreme cases, sufferers may lie fully awake until two or three o'clock in the morning. They want to sleep, but their systems refuse to let them sleep because their timing is disrupted.

The opposite is a sleep disorder known as advanced sleep phase syndrome, in which victims become fatigued and sleepy much earlier than they should, sometimes as early as seven or eight o'clock in the evening. Because they tend to fall asleep at such an early hour, victims of advance sleep phase syndrome often wake up in the early hours of the morning—long before they would like. This particular problem is a common complaint among older people.

Rarer still and extremely difficult to deal with is what sleep researchers call the non-24-hour sleep/wake cycle, which causes its victims to stay awake for an extended period and then plunges them into a deep sleep for an equally long period. In extreme cases this disorder can result in a sleep/wake cycle that is 48 hours or more in length.

As you might imagine, being so out-of-sync with the rest of the world can be extremely problematic. Those who can't fall asleep until the wee hours of the morning often find themselves physically exhausted as they struggle to work a normal nine-to-five shift. And those who fall asleep early and awaken long before morning frequently lack any semblance of an evening social life because they can't keep their eyes open past 8 PM or so. It's a frustrating, often agonizing way to live and as a result the victims of such sleep disorders are often overstressed and depressed.

## How are sleep problems caused by disrupted circadian rhythms typically treated?

Many sleep disorders resulting from disrupted circadian rhythms can be corrected through a technique known as chronotherapy. This process uses brief exposure to bright light to reset the body's internal clock and make it function on a more normal schedule. Researchers still do not fully understand how chronotherapy works, although one possible answer is that light helps regulate the production of sleep-inducing brain hormones such as melatonin.

**I'm seeing a doctor for help in alleviating my insomnia. My doctor told me that there are actually several distinct types of this sleep disorder. Is this true?**

Clinically speaking, yes. The layperson's use of the word insomnia is usually an umbrella phrase for an inability to get to sleep or stay asleep. But sleep researchers divide insomnia into a number of different classifications based on specific symptoms and other factors that help to identify the cause of the insomnia. The cause is important because it can play an important role in determining treatment.

Doctors typically subdivide generalized insomnia into three categories: difficulty falling asleep (known clinically as sleep onset or initial insomnia), frequent or lengthy awakenings during the night (sleep maintenance or middle insomnia), early morning awakening with the inability to return to sleep (terminal insomnia), or fatigue during the day even after a full night's sleep (nonrestorative sleep).

Insomnia lasting one day to several days is known as transient insomnia and is most commonly caused by daily stress or a change in environment. Difficulty sleeping, which may last from a few days to three weeks, is known as short-term insomnia and is typically caused by stressful situations such as a serious illness, getting fired, or divorce. Insomnia lasting months or years is called long-term or chronic insomnia and may be caused by psychiatric or health problems, the use of certain medications, or a primary sleep disorder.

**What kinds of primary sleep disorders can result in long-term insomnia?**

There are several. Psychophysiological insomnia is a behavioral problem characterized by a preoccupation with one's inability to fall asleep. It is often triggered initially by a stressful situation, but sleep difficulties persist long after the stress has disappeared. Many people with this condition worry so much about their inability to fall asleep that it becomes a self-fulfilling prophecy, or a conditioned response. Most people with psychophysiological insomnia find that they have little difficulty falling asleep when they're not really trying—when taking a Saturday afternoon nap, for example, or when they go on vacation. In most cases, people with psychophysiological insomnia find fast relief through behavioral therapy and/or relaxation training.

A sleep problem triggered by outside factors such as an unfamiliar environment is known as adjustment sleep disorder or transient situational insomnia. It can occur when someone finds themselves in a strange new bed (in a hotel, for example) or following a major life event, such as loss of a loved one or starting a new job. Most cases of adjustment sleep disorder disappear on their own within a couple of weeks.

A related disorder, known as inadequate sleep hygiene, can occur when an individual becomes excited or hyperactive just before bedtime, or is in an environment that just is not conducive to sleep. The most common problems include too much light or noise in the bedroom, extremes in temperature, or a bed that is too soft or too hard. Sleep researchers say the answer is to develop a bedtime ritual conducive to sleep (a soothing bath, quiet music, a massage, aroma therapy), to eliminate environmental problems, and to use the bedroom only for sleep and not for reading, eating, or watching television.

Another common sleep disturbance is altitude insomnia, which is just as its name describes—an inability to fall asleep at high altitudes. Common characteristics include slowed, periodic breathing (apnea), frequent awakenings, and generally poor quality of sleep. Altitude insomnia usually lasts just a few days, but it can persist longer in sensitive individuals. Taking medications that facilitate a sound, deep sleep is often beneficial.

Insomnia is also often triggered by specific drugs. Caffeine—a powerful stimulant—is one of the most common offenders. Sensitive individuals who consume coffee or other caffeine-rich foods or beverages prior to bedtime may find sleep all but impossible. And when they finally do fall asleep, it's seldom restful. Many people have a cup of coffee with dinner, not realizing that the effects of the caffeine they are consuming can affect their system for several hours afterward.

Alcohol—often used to induce sleep—can have a rebound effect resulting in increased awakenings and generally poor slumber. People with sleep apnea, a disorder characterized by loud snoring and impaired breathing, should avoid alcohol before bedtime because it tends to make the condition even worse.

Drugs such as cocaine and amphetamines can also dramatically affect one's ability to fall sleep and sleep soundly. So can withdrawal from certain sedatives and sleeping pills, a condition known as rebound insomnia.

**Can depression play a role in the onset of insomnia? A good friend has been depressed ever since her daughter was stillborn, and she often complains of her inability to get a good night's sleep.**

Your friend sounds like a textbook case of depression-related sleep disruption. In fact, sleep disturbances are a common symptom of depression, including sleep onset insomnia, sleep maintenance insomnia, and early morning wakefulness. However, many depressed people, especially adolescents and those afflicted with bipolar or seasonal affective disorder (SAD), experience the opposite extreme and sleep all the time.

Studies show that insomnia can be a predictive factor for the onset of a depressive episode. In fact, you may have trouble sleeping long before you or your family and friends notice any substantial change in your mood. By the same token, insomnia often disappears as the depressive episode starts to wane. In many cases, the use of antidepressant medication can improve both mood and sleep function.

## Is narcolepsy a side effect of insomnia?

No. Narcolepsy is a bizarre and relatively uncommon sleep disorder characterized by extreme daytime sleepiness, sudden and involuntary episodes of daytime sleep, disturbed nighttime sleep, and sudden weakness of muscle tone (known as cataplexy), which is often triggered by intense emotion. Many people also report paralysis and hallucinations at the onset of sleep or upon awakening. The duration of a narcoleptic attack can range from just a few seconds of transient paralysis to paralysis of the entire body lasting 20 minutes or longer in extreme cases.

Approximately 200,000 Americans suffer from narcolepsy to varying degrees; some experience episodes almost daily, while others may experience one every few months or even years. Clinical studies suggest a genetic connection to the disorder, with first-degree relatives of narcoleptics commonly demonstrating excessive daytime sleepiness and a noticeably higher incidence of narcolepsy than in the general public.

The symptoms of narcolepsy usually begin when someone is in their 20s, although researchers have seen cases that began as young as 5 years old and as old as 50. In many cases, severe stress such as divorce or the loss of a loved one immediately precedes onset of the condition. Thankfully, the majority of cases of narcolepsy can be adequately controlled with medication, including mild stimulants to counter sleepiness and antidepressants for associated cataplexy, hallucinations, and sleep paralysis.

## Is there a connection between snoring and sleep disturbances?

Yes, a very strong one. Sleep apnea, for example, is a condition characterized by wall-shaking snoring and obstructed breathing that can interfere with your sleep all night long (not to mention that of anyone sleeping next to you). Sleep apnea is most commonly seen in overweight men and seniors and is closely linked to hypertension (high blood pressure). However, sleep apnea doesn't discriminate; people who are slight of build and even children can suffer with it night after night.

In severe cases of sleep apnea, victims may stop breathing for as long as a minute and a half before startling themselves awake. Not surprisingly, many sleep apnea patients report feeling fatigued, confused, and unable to think clearly throughout the day even though they think they've had a good night's sleep. In truth, people with sleep apnea awaken themselves dozens, even hundreds of times each night, which prevents them from successfully going through the many stages of sleep necessary to feel rested and refreshed in the morning. Worse still, sleep apnea has also been linked to increased risk of serious illness including heart disease and early death. Luckily, most types of sleep apnea can be successfully treated.

**My husband is constantly jiggling his legs, even in bed at night as he's trying to go to sleep. He hasn't slept well in a long time, and I think his restless legs are part of the reason why. Should he see a doctor?**

You should consult a qualified sleep disorder specialist anytime you have extended periods of insomnia or other sleep disturbances, especially if lack of sleep is affecting your physical and mental health.

Your husband may suffer from a condition known as restless legs syndrome, which is signaled by an irresistible urge to move one's legs, especially when inactive. Most sufferers report a sensation similar to something crawling deep within their calves or thighs and say it can be relieved only by movement. Severity may increase or decrease over a period of months or years, and the disorder can be triggered by a number of factors including caffeine, an iron deficiency, and pregnancy. Approximately 12 percent of insomnia patients seen at sleep clinics have restless legs syndrome to some degree.

Many people with this condition jiggle their legs while lying in bed waiting for sleep to come, and they may periodically jiggle their legs after they fall asleep, which can be extremely irritating to their bed mates. Not surprisingly, victims of restless legs syndrome are often drowsy during the day because their condition prevents them from getting a night of satisfying, restful sleep. Treatment options for restless legs syndrome are limited, although many patients respond well to therapy with medications such as clonazepam (Klonopin) or a combination of carbidopa and levodopa (Sinemet).

## Can insomnia and related sleep disorders be caused by specific medical conditions?

Absolutely. Quite a few medical conditions have been associated with sleep problems, although some of these sleep disturbances may result indirectly from the medical condition, such as poor sleep as a result of chronic pain from arthritis or fibromyalgia.

The detrimental effect on sleep is more pronounced with other medical conditions, however. Asthma, for example, can be especially problematic because related breathing difficulties at night can make sleep difficult. Experts note that common treatments for asthma, such as adrenergic agonists and glucocorticoids, can also disrupt sleep. An effective alternative is inhaled steroids, which do not typically affect sleep.

Heart specialists say that poor blood supply to the heart, a condition called cardiac ischemia, can also have a profound effect on sleep. It is not uncommon for people afflicted with this condition to experience bouts of angina (chest pain due to inadequate blood flow to or through the coronary arteries that supply blood to the heart) while sleeping. They are also more prone to disturbing dreams and nightmares, although researchers are unsure why.

Emphysema, also called chronic obstructive pulmonary disease (COPD), is very common among seniors, especially those who smoke, and has long been associated with sleep difficulties. Poor breathing is the primary culprit, a problem often exacerbated by sleeping in a flat position. Many COPD patients report improved sleep when lying semi-upright.

Other conditions commonly associated with disrupted sleep patterns include depression, cystic fibrosis, hyperthyroidism, kidney disease, menopause, pregnancy, enlarged prostate (prostatic hypertrophy), uterine prolapse, liver disease, and gastroesophageal reflux.

## My wife is pregnant, and has been having trouble sleeping for several weeks. Is this normal?

Yes. Insomnia is a common complaint among pregnant women and it has many causes. As a baby grows and bears increasing weight on a woman's bladder, she often finds that she needs to urinate with greater frequency. Unfortunately, this means frequent trips to the bathroom in the middle of the night, which in turn can prevent her from getting a good night's sleep. Pregnancy can also stimulate bizarre and very vivid dreams, which may interfere with normal sleep patterns. And as a pregnant woman's stomach grows larger, she may find it increasingly difficult to find a comfortable sleep position.

As any mother will tell you, the sleep situation hardly improves once a baby is born, especially if the new arrival is being breast-fed. Late-night feedings, diaper changes, daily care, visiting friends, and new-mom anxiety all conspire to take up every free moment a woman has. As a result, pregnancy-related insomnia gives way to plain old exhaustion as the new mother struggles to do everything that must be done when a new child is brought home. And things change little as a child grows up. Most mothers, even those who work outside the home, wear many hats around the house and struggle to take care of innumerable daily chores and family obligations that rob them of energy and force them to stay up late and get up early.

Unlike other people who suffer from sleep disorders, pregnant and breast-feeding women usually cannot turn to medication to help them sleep because of potential side effects to their babies. But that doesn't mean a pregnant woman has to suffer. Nonpharmacological alternatives to better sleep include a warm bath and a massage before bedtime (this is also a great way for new parents to spend a little quality time together at night), stress-reducing music, and soothing herbal teas. However, you should consult your doctor before consuming any herbal compound to make sure it's safe for pregnant women. Many are not.

## I'm approaching the age of menopause. Should I expect some sleep problems as my body adjusts to the change of life?

All women react differently to menopause, but insomnia and disrupted sleep are common complaints among many menopausal women. Like pregnancy, the physical changes experienced by a woman undergoing menopause are the most likely culprit. Hot flashes, for example, can awaken you in the middle of the night, drenching your body in sweat no matter how cool the room. Some menopausal women never experience hot flashes while others are awakened by them several times a night. The body's rapidly falling estrogen levels can also promote fatigue, depression, and other conditions that may adversely affect a woman's quality of sleep. Hormone replacement therapy can often make menopause easier to bear.

## How do sleep specialists evaluate and diagnose insomnia?

There are a number of tests for determining the extent and possible causes of chronic insomnia or related sleep disorders. One test, known as the Multiple Sleep Latency Test, measures how long it takes a person to fall asleep in a darkened room—that is, under normal sleep conditions. The length of time can vary dramatically depending on what kind of sleep disorder a person has and how long the person has been afflicted. Healthy individuals usually fall asleep within 20 minutes, but those who are extremely fatigued may drop off in less than 5 minutes, and those with chronic insomnia may lie awake for hours even though they desperately crave sleep.

Sleep clinics, which are often associated with major teaching hospitals and universities, rely on a number of medical disciplines including neurology, psychiatry, and cardiology to evaluate, diagnose, and treat sleep disorders. Their goal is to determine if there is a medical or psychiatric cause for the problem. If none is readily apparent, patients may be asked to spend one or more nights at the clinic so specialists can monitor their electrical brain activity, eye movements, and other physiologic responses during sleep. Sleep clinics are not inexpensive, but for a lot of insomnia patients they are the hope of last resort. Thankfully, sleep clinics are very adept at finding the cause of a person's sleep difficulty, no matter how unusual.

## I suffer from occasional insomnia. Could you offer some tips on how to maintain healthy sleep patterns and keep insomnia from occurring in the first place?

Most insomnia can be relieved with medication, but there are a number of ways to facilitate a good night's sleep without having to resort to medication. The following are good ways to establish and maintain healthy sleep patterns.

- **Reduce stress and anxiety in your life.** Stress is one of the biggest causes of transient insomnia because it keeps the brain awake and functioning long after it should have closed up shop for the night. Stress causes worry, and worry interferes with sleep. Acknowledging the problem is the first step, followed by a resolution to take care of those problems you can, and a promise not to dwell on those you cannot. See Chapter 2: Stress and Anxiety for more advice on how to keep stress and anxiety from ruling your life and preventing you from getting enough sleep.

- **Maintain a healthy lifestyle.** This means eating right and getting enough exercise. But sleep specialists warn that you should not exercise immediately before bedtime. Physical activity tends to stimulate the body rather than relax it. It is better to exercise first thing in the morning or shortly after you get home from work. Save the evening for relaxation.

- **Establish a sleep schedule.** Determine the best time for you to go to sleep (it's different for everyone and depends on how much sleep you need to feel rested and alert the next day) and try to hit the sack at exactly that time every evening. A soothing bedtime ritual can also help.

- **Use your bed for sleep only—not for eating, watching television, or reading.** Those are activities that should be done anywhere but in the bedroom. The goal is to quickly prepare your body for sleep when you finally go to bed.

- **Make sure your bed is comfortable, including your pillow.** A bed that is too hard or too soft can have a serious effect on your ability to fall asleep and stay asleep. When shopping for a new mattress, check out as many different kinds as you can before making your decision. Never buy the first mattress you see. And never buy a mattress without lying on it for several minutes to determine how it feels.

- **Make sure your bedroom is conducive to sleep.** Many people sleep poorly because their bedrooms are too noisy, too bright, too hot, or too cold. Some people can sleep under almost any conditions, but most of us need darkness and comfort for a truly good night's sleep. Consider soundproofing if outside noise fills your bedroom, and blackout curtains to keep out light. And don't forget the small stuff. Even something as inconsequential as a bright clock face can inhibit sleep in sensitive individuals.

- **Don't linger in bed when the alarm clock goes off.** Hitting the snooze button again and again can have a detrimental effect on your internal clock and make you feel fatigued and fuzzy-brained all day long. Establishing a set time to get up each morning keeps your body clock in sync and helps ensure restful sleep.

- **Resist the occasional afternoon nap.** It may seem like a good idea, but naps usually just interfere with your nighttime sleep patterns.

- **Avoid alcohol and tobacco.** Alcohol may make you drowsy, but it interferes with brain activity and actually impairs sleep. And nicotine is a powerful stimulant—the last thing you need if you're having trouble falling asleep.

- **Skip that late-night snack.** A stomach full of fried chicken or chocolate cake can interfere with sleep by forcing your body to work when it should be resting. In addition, heavy, greasy foods can trigger indigestion, which will definitely keep you from enjoying a good night's sleep.

- **Don't lie awake in bed if you have trouble falling asleep right away.** After 15 or 20 minutes, get up and do something. Read a book or listen to soft music—anything to relax and ease you toward sleep. If you have trouble falling asleep but usually sleep well when your eyes finally close, readjust your sleep schedule and go to bed a little later.

**I travel overseas frequently and find that jet lag greatly interferes with my ability to get a good night's sleep once I reach my destination. Sometimes it takes me two or three days to reestablish a healthy sleep pattern. Is there anything I can do to alleviate this problem?**

Jet lag is a common cause of sleep difficulties, but there are ways to minimize its effects and possibly prevent it from bothering you. For example, make sure you drink a lot of water over the course of a lengthy flight to avoid dehydration from high altitudes and changes in air pressure. Also, avoid alcohol and caffeine, both of which can adversely affect your sleep cycle. If you exercise regularly at home, try to maintain your schedule at your new destination even if it's something as simple as taking a brisk walk around the block. Inactivity can play a big role in promoting poor sleep. Finally, try to eat the three big meals of the day on local time rather than on home time (despite what your stomach says). This will help your brain adjust more quickly to the time change and promote a good night's sleep.

**My doctor wants to put me on a short course of medication to help ease my sleeping problems. What kinds of medications are most often used in the treatment of insomnia, and how effective are they?**

Medication can be very effective in treating both transient and chronic insomnia, and you would do well to follow your doctor's advice if nonpharmacological approaches have not helped.

There are a number of over-the-counter sleep aids for occasional nights of sleeplessness, including Sominex, Sleep-Eze, and Unisom. Most of these compounds contain antihistamines such as diphenhydramine or doxylamine to promote drowsiness. These chemicals are also the active ingredients in many over-the-counter allergy medications, which is why you should never drive or operate heavy machinery when under their influence.

Nonprescription sleep aids can be somewhat expensive, so you might want to buy a generic antihistamine product instead. The result will be the same, and you'll save a few dollars in the process. Some newer antihistamines contain nondrowsy formulas, so make sure you buy the kind that will definitely put you to sleep.

A warning: Antihistamines can be effective in easing occasional transient insomnia, but they should not be used to treat chronic sleeplessness. They should also not be used by people with certain chronic illnesses such as glaucoma, asthma, seizures, and benign prostatic hypertrophy. Antihistamines can also trigger a number of side effects besides drowsiness including dry mouth and rapid heartbeat, and they often leave you feeling dried out and hungover upon awakening. If you are afflicted with a chronic illness, consult your doctor before taking over-the-counter antihistamines.

If nonprescription products don't do the trick, your doctor may prescribe one of the many benzodiazepine sedative/hypnotics, such as diazepam (Valium), alprazolam (Xanax), clorazepate (Tranxene), or temazepam (Restoril). These medications are especially useful in easing insomnia due to generalized anxiety, and they are far safer than barbiturates. However, they are far from perfect. As discussed earlier in this book, benzodiazepine use can produce a number of side effects and, over an extended period, can lead to dependence. They also suppress the dream stage of sleep, resulting in what are known as "rebound nightmares" in certain individuals. Benzodiazepines can also react adversely when mixed with alcohol.

Several antidepressants prescribed in low doses may also be helpful in promoting better sleep, especially in people whose sleep disorders are caused by situational depression, such as depression that results from the death of a loved one, divorce, or loss of a job. Some of the most commonly prescribed medications in this family include amitriptyline (Elavil), trazodone (Desyrel), amoxapine (Asendin), and doxepin (Sinequan). These medications help promote slumber without affecting dream states, but there can be other uncomfortable side effects, including dry mouth and a feeling of confusion or fuzzy thinking upon awakening.

A non-benzodiazepine sedative/hypnotic, zolpidem (Ambien), has recently become available. This medication has been approved for the short-term treatment of insomnia. It has a number of advantages over the benzodiazepines because it reportedly lacks potential for abuse or dependence and does not produce hangover effects or promote daytime sedation. Zolpidem has been approved for short-term use only, and studies investigating long-term use are currently under way.

The upside to therapy with medications is that it can help people suffering from insomnia fall asleep. The downside is that many medications can affect the type and quality of sleep you get. Benzodiazepines, for example, are known to affect various phases of sleep and reduce the amount of time you spend in dream states. This can, in extreme cases, affect memory and result in physical and psychiatric problems. In addition, long-term use of certain sleep aids can actually make you resistant to their sleep-promoting effects, requiring ever-increasing doses to achieve the same end.

If your doctor suggests benzodiazepines to help you sleep, ask about duration of use (benzodiazepines should *not* be used to treat chronic, long-term insomnia, although many doctors prescribe it for this purpose anyway) and potential side effects. If you don't like the answers, discuss alternatives—including the use of kava and other herbal therapies. See Chapter 5: Treating Insomnia with Kava and Other Remedies for more information on alternatives to treating insomnia with medications.

# FOUR

## Treating Stress and Anxiety with Kava and Other Remedies

*FACT:* Kava is not a new stress-busting phenomenon. The South Pacific islanders have used kava to ease stress and anxiety for centuries, and kava-based medicines have been available in Europe since the 1880s.

*FACT:* Numerous clinical studies in Germany and elsewhere have confirmed that kava is as effective as many prescription sedatives when it comes to reducing the effects of stress and anxiety.

*FACT:* Kava is so widely regarded in Germany that doctors often prescribe it for anxiety as a first line of treatment before turning to benzodiazepines and other medications.

*FACT:* Kava isn't the only effective herbal stress buster on the market. Others include St. John's Wort, valerian, passionflower, and hops (not the kind used to make beer). All work well—and with few side effects.

*Remember Betty, our overworked, overstressed midlevel corporate executive in Chapter 1? Not long after Betty's Day From Hell, she had a visit from her friend Sharon, a 36-year-old postal employee whose well-paying job carries a lot of stress. Sharon usually handled her job with amazing aplomb, taking care of problems as they occurred and refusing to let stress and anxiety run her life. But one day Sharon came knocking on Betty's door, distraught, shaking, and anxious. The stress she had been handling so well had suddenly become overwhelming, to the point where Sharon was seriously considering changing careers.*

*Betty took Sharon out to dinner and listened attentively as her good friend cited a litany of work-related problems that threatened to plunge her into a nervous breakdown. She had started drinking a lot of wine after work to help her cope, and her relationship with her boyfriend was in turmoil over her unpredictable moods. Back at Betty's apartment, Sharon asked for a glass of wine to take the edge off, but Betty shook her head. "I have something better," she said. "An herbal tea that will calm you down, improve your thinking, and even help you sleep."*

*It sounded too good to be true, but Sharon agreed to try kava. It tasted odd even with a dash of honey, but she downed one cup and then another. Within an hour Sharon felt calmer than she had in weeks. She also really felt like talking, so she and Betty discussed at length Sharon's problems at work and with her boyfriend, as well as possible solutions. By the end of the evening, Sharon was actually looking forward to going to work the next day.*

*Sharon is now a kava convert. She keeps kava powder and tablets in her kitchen pantry and turns to them instead of wine to calm down at the end of an especially hard day. "I'm certain that kava saved me from becoming either an alcoholic or a tranquilizer junkie," Sharon says. "I don't use it every day, just when the stress starts to get to me. It calms me down and I feel great the next day. I can't say enough good things about the stuff. I even have my boyfriend drinking it!"*

Betty and Sharon are part of a growing "kava movement" that is taking the United States by storm. Every year, more and more Americans discover what the South Pacific islanders and many Europeans have known for years: Kava is a safe and effective remedy for the stress and anxiety of our workaday world. It relaxes and calms without causing fuzzy or impaired thinking, and several studies have found kava to be considerably safer than prescription sedatives.

In this chapter, we'll discuss the best ways to treat stress and anxiety with kava, the many international clinical studies that have confirmed its usefulness, and other natural stress busters available in most neighborhood grocery and health food stores.

## We know that the South Pacific islanders have used kava medicinally for hundreds, perhaps thousands of years. How recent is the medicinal use of the plant among westerners?

Europeans and Americans have not used kava as a medicinal herb nearly as long as the residents of Oceania, but it is incorrect to think that westerners have only recently discovered the plant's amazing curative properties. Kava-based pills and syrups have been in use as far back as the late 1880s and were commonly recommended by German herbalists. By the turn of the century preparations containing kava were being offered by British doctors for the treatment of a number of ailments, and in 1914 kava was finally listed in the *British Pharmacopoeia* under the name kava rhizoma. By 1920, kava was being used throughout much of Europe as a sedative and a blood pressure treatment. Around that time, the herb was also being promoted in the United States Dispensory as a remedy for chronic urinary infections, and by 1950 it was frequently prescribed in the United States under the names Gonosan and Neurocardin as a treatment for gonorrhea and nervous disorders, including anxiety.

**How common is the use of kava in Europe today?**

Very common. Kava is used medicinally in several European countries, most notably Switzerland, France, the United Kingdom, and Germany, where a number of impressive studies have been conducted on the herb. In fact, it's estimated that nearly 100 tons of kava are imported into Europe annually for the manufacture of tinctures, pills, and capsules.

**Please discuss some of the more important clinical studies that have confirmed kava's effectiveness as a treatment for stress and anxiety.**

Many studies have been done on kava over the years, but one of the most impressive—and conclusive—was conducted in 1997 by Dr. Hans-Peter Volz, a researcher in the Department of Psychiatry at Jena University in Germany, and Dr. M. Kieser, a researcher with the German pharmaceutical company Dr. Willmar Schwabe GmbH, which manufactures a widely used standardized kava extract known as WS 1490. The placebo-controlled study involved 101 anxiety patients at ten medical centers throughout the southern part of Germany and sought to establish the safety and efficacy of the herb in the treatment of anxiety conditions. All of the participants suffered from anxiety and tension, though many had other complications, including agoraphobia, specific phobia, and adjustment disorder with anxiety. Patients with extreme medical or psychological problems were excluded from the study, and participants were given numerous psychological assessments, including the Hamilton Anxiety Scale and the Adjective Mood Scale, to establish their mental status and severity of anxiety prior to and throughout the study.

The subjects were divided into two groups. One group received a placebo (a sugar pill) three times a day, while the other group was given concentrated kava extract containing about 70 milligrams of active kavalactones three times daily. The study lasted 25 weeks, and the results were impressive. Not surprisingly, both the short-term and long-term effectiveness of kava was much greater than the placebo. Most patients showed a marked improvement in symptoms within eight weeks, and the effectiveness of the herb improved dramatically as the study progressed. The most noticeable improvements were seen in anxious mood, tension, fear, and sleeplessness. After 24 weeks, 75 percent of the kava recipients showed definite improvements as compared to only 51 percent of those given a placebo.

The researchers also noted that those in the kava group seemed to tolerate the herb very well, and few side effects or adverse reactions were noted. Analysis of various body systems and functions including heart rate, blood pressure, red and white blood cell counts, liver enzymes, and blood sugar showed that none were affected by kava.

Volz and Kieser concluded: "These results support (kava) as a treatment alternative to tricyclic antidepressants and benzodiazepines in anxiety disorders, with proven long-term efficacy and none of the tolerance problems associated with tricyclics and benzodiazepines."

There have been a number of other kava studies as well, although none as lengthy as the one conducted by Volz and Kieser. In 1991, for example, researchers at the Gerontopsychiatry Center in Dusseldorf, Germany, conducted a double-blind, placebo-controlled study of kava involving 29 patients suffering from anxiety. Participants received either 100 milligrams of WS 1490 kava extract (70 milligrams kavalactones per capsule) three times a day or a placebo equivalent. Like the Volz-Kieser study, benefits were noted right from the start. Many subjects reported improvement within one week and continued improvement over the course of the four-week study. Again, no serious side effects were noted and the subjects appeared to tolerate the kava quite well.

A more recent four-week, double-blind study conducted by German researchers in 1996 showed similar results.

Fifty-eight patients, all afflicted with anxiety problems, were given either a placebo or kava extract containing 70 percent kavalactones three times a day. Those receiving kava reported a noticeable reduction in anxiety with no side effects.

## What are the most prominent benefits of kava when the herb is compared to commonly pre- scribed commercial anxiolytics?

There are many, and most have been confirmed by clin- ical research. For example, kava does not interfere with memory or mental function the way benzodiazepines can, nor is it physiologically addictive. In addition, researchers have found that there are no symptoms of withdrawal when someone stops taking kava (as compared to the agitation, sleeplessness, potential seizures, and other health problems that can arise when someone stops taking benzodiazepines), nor have there been any reports of death or serious illness stemming from normal use of the herb. Best of all, the effectiveness of kava does not taper off over time. Certain prescription medications may require a gradual increase in dosage to maintain efficacy, but kava remains effective at a standard dose no matter how long you take it.

On the other side of the coin, kava is often less effective in treating the symptoms of severe stress and anxiety and has little effect on anxiety-related agitation. It is a trade-off, but for mild to moderate anxiety disorders, kava can be an effective first-line treatment.

## Have researchers ever monitored the brain waves of people taking kava? It seems to me that could be a good way of evaluating the plant's mental and physiological effects.

Researchers in the Department of Psychiatry at the University of Vienna, Austria, did just that in the late 1980s in a landmark study on kawain (also known as kavain), one of the most potent kavalactones. Eight men and seven women, all in good mental and physical health, randomly received a placebo, kawain in strengths ranging from 200 to 600 milligrams, or 30 milligrams of clobazam (Frisium), a benzodiazepine used as a reference dose. The brain waves of the subjects were monitored via an electroencephalograph (EEG) at the time the dose was given and again one, two, four, six, and eight hours later. Psychological tests were also administered and side effects, if any, were recorded.

The EEG showed a significant change in brain wave activity in the subjects receiving kawain. In fact, the greater the amount consumed, the slower their brain wave activity. The researchers reported that a noticeable increase in theta and delta waves and a decrease in beta waves—all of which help induce the onset of relaxing sleep—was most evident at the 200 milligram dose of kawain. The subjects were also most alert at doses of 200 milligrams, with higher doses causing more sedation.

More startling was the comparison of kavain and clobazam when subjects were asked to perform psychological tests. Those on kava experienced a noticeable improvement in intellectual performance regardless of dose, while those given clobazam reported just the opposite.

The effects of pure kava extract on brain wave activity are a little different from those seen in people receiving just kawain. In one revealing study, two healthy men and five healthy women were given kava extract daily for a week, followed by a week in which they were kava-free. A placebo group showed no changes in brain wave patterns, but those who had received kava had EEG results similar to those seen in people taking sedative/hypnotic drugs: specifically an increase in beta waves and a decrease in alpha waves. However, unlike kawain, kava did not stimulate sleep-promoting delta and theta waves. The researchers also determined through a process known as event-related potential studies that kava helps the brain process information better by improving concentration and attention to detail.

Bottom line: Kava has a psychoactive profile similar to that of commonly prescribed anxiolytics but without the unwanted side effects. It eases anxiety just as effectively, but it does not cloud thinking, concentration, or perception like some prescription medications can do. This was demonstrated in a recent double-blind (a test in which neither doctors nor study participants know who is getting the medication as opposed to placebo) German study in which 38 patients with anxiety-related problems were treated with either kawain and a placebo for oxazepam (Serax) or oxazepam and a placebo for kawain. Subjects were given either a 200 milligram capsule of kawain three times a day along with the placebo for oxazepam twice a day or a 10 milligram tablet of oxazepam twice a day plus the placebo for kawain three times a day. The effectiveness of the compounds were determined using the Anxiety Status Inventory and the Zung Self-Rating Anxiety Scale.

At the end of the study it was determined that anxiety symptoms in both groups, as measured by the two scales, decreased by an average of 65 percent. The conclusion: Kawain is just as beneficial as oxazepam in helping many anxiety patients.

### Have any studies looked at the effects of kava on simple anxiety problems that are not psychiatric in origin?

Yes. In 1996, Dr. E. Lehmann and colleagues published a report on such a study in the journal *Phytomedicine*. Fifty-eight subjects with anxiety syndromes determined not to be caused by mental disorders were divided into two groups. One group received 100 milligrams of standardized kava extract three times a day for four weeks, and the second group received a placebo equivalent. A variety of assessments, including the Hamilton Anxiety Scale, were used to evaluate anxiety in both groups. The clear winner was kava: Subjects receiving the herb showed significantly lower anxiety scores than those receiving the placebo. The re-searchers noted that the herb worked remarkably fast, with many subjects reporting noticeable improvement in anxiety and tension levels after just one week. By the end of the study, almost all of the subjects receiving kava said they felt less anxiety, less nervousness, and a greater sense of well-being.

Another study examined the impact of kava on the daily stress and anxiety of adults who did not have a clinical anxiety condition. Dr. Y. N. Singh and his research group performed a double-blind placebo-controlled study in 60 adults with elevated levels of daily stress and anxiety. Participants were treated for four weeks with either one kava capsule twice a day (60 kavalactones per capsule) or a placebo equivalent. Responses were measured using several assessment scales including the Daily Stress Inventory and the State-Trait Anxiety Inventory. Dr. Singh found that, yet again, kava came out on top. The herb was found to reduce the stress associated with the daily hassles of life including interpersonal problems, personal competency, worries, environmental stresses, and other varied problems. These results were not seen in individuals taking a placebo. Further reductions were observed with longer use of the herb.

**I'm menopausal, and I experience a low level of anxiety on a regular basis. Have there been any studies regarding the effects of kava on this and other menopause-related problems? I'd rather take something natural like kava than a prescription medication that might cause side effects.**

Again, we have to turn to Germany for the kind of clinical research you are asking about. In 1991, a German gynecologist named G. Warnecke studied the effects of kava in 40 women between ages 45 to 60 who were experiencing a number of menopausal symptoms, including anxiety. Twenty subjects received a 100 milligram capsule of standardized kava extract three times a day for two months while the other group received placebo. The effects of the herb versus placebo were measured using a variety of tests, including the Hamilton Anxiety Scale, the Depression Status Inventory, and the Kupperman Index, which gauges the severity of menopausal symptoms.

The beneficial effects of kava were dramatic, Dr. Warnecke noted in the German medical journal *Fortschritte der Medizin*. Most of the women receiving kava experienced a 50 percent reduction in anxiety symptoms within the first week of the study and reported almost no anxiety at all by the end of the first month. Kava also helped reduce the severity of a number of other menopausal symptoms including depressive moodiness, restlessness, and irritability. By the end of the study, many of the women receiving kava said they felt better than they had in months, while those receiving a placebo reported little change in their menopausal symptoms.

Here in the United States, a growing number of menopausal women are turning to kava to help ease the symptoms of menopause. "I was a wreck before a friend suggested I try kava," notes Kate, a 52-year-old executive secretary. "I felt anxious and tense all the time, and hot flashes would awaken me in a drenching sweat almost every night. In addition, my family and coworkers couldn't stand to be around me because I was constantly irritable and moody. I can't blame them—I didn't like me very much either. But after two weeks of taking kava every day, my symptoms became much more tolerable. They didn't disappear completely, but they were mild enough that I could live with them. I later started hormone replacement therapy on the advice of my gynecologist, but kava definitely helped me over the worst of my menopause."

**It seems that the majority of clinical studies on kava have taken place in Germany. Is the herb widely used there?**

Most definitely—and with the approval of Commission E, a unique government agency similar to our Food and Drug Administration that approves effective herbs as over-the-counter medications.

Kava is so highly regarded in Germany as a remedy for symptoms of stress and anxiety that doctors there often prescribe it to patients and insurance companies usually pick up the bill. More than 350,000 kava prescriptions are written in Germany annually, resulting in about $14 million (US) in sales.

**All of this talk about the beneficial effects of kava on stress, anxiety, and other disorders has me ready to give it a try. But how much should I take? What's the recommended dosage?**

Numerous factors influence the amount of kava you should take including the problem you are taking it for, your age, and— most importantly—your sensitivity to the herb's effects. Some people react well to just a little bit of kava, while others need a stronger dose.

As with any medicinal product, whether it is a prescription medication or a natural herb, it is always best to start with a small dose and then increase it if necessary. By proceeding slowly, you will minimize any potential side effects or adverse reactions, although in general kava has proven quite safe for most people.

If you have never tried kava before, most herbalists suggest starting with a daily capsule containing between 60 to 70 milligrams of kavalactones, although some experts recommend a higher beginning dose. Most commercial kava products have dosage information on the label or in the accompanying literature. Take the capsule on an evening when you have no plans, so you can enjoy and evaluate the herb's effects without having to worry about work, driving, or operating heavy machinery. Taking kava in the evening is also recommended because in some sensitive individuals kava can result in drowsiness.

If you have a sensitive constitution, a single kava capsule should produce the desired results: a feeling of calm and tranquility as stress melts from your body, and an overall sensation of relaxation. However, if you do not feel anything after one capsule, try two capsules the following evening if needed. If again you feel nothing, gradually increase your dosage over the next few days until you get the effects you are seeking. Most people feel the influence of kava when they have taken between 70 to 140 milligrams of kavalactones, but in more severe cases of stress or anxiety even higher levels may be required to achieve therapeutic results. In cases such as these, some people find it more effective to take one to two capsules two to three times a day.

Kava is generally regarded as safe, but there is always a very small risk that it could interact negatively with other medications or an extremely sensitive system. If any adverse reactions are experienced as a result of taking kava, discontinue use and consider other soothing herbs instead.

## What's the most effective way to take kava?

Kava is available in the United States in pill, capsule, tincture (liquid), and powder form. The best way to take it depends on you. Most people like the ease of pills, but some prefer making a beverage out of the powder or liquid, although the taste can be off-putting and may take some getting used to. Make sure you read the label of the product you buy to ensure you are getting quality kava extract with sufficient quantities of kavalactones. We will discuss the different forms of kava and their purchase in greater detail in Chapter 7: Shopping for Kava.

## Do the natives of the South Pacific islands who drink kava ingest the same amount of kavalactones as I do when I take a commercial product?

They probably consume considerably more. One study of kava done in Fiji found that the average cup or coconut shell of the elixir contained about 250 milligrams of kavalactones, and it is safe to assume that more potent forms of kava produced elsewhere in the region contain even higher levels. It is not beyond the realm of possibility for a South Pacific islander to consume as much as 2,000 milligrams of kavalactones drinking kava over the course of an evening. However, we obviously do not need that much to achieve a pleasant state of tranquility and relaxation.

## Will taking kava prevent me from driving or doing my job? I don't want to take it if it's going to zonk me out to the point where I can't function.

Kava does not impair thinking, concentration, or memory in the vast majority of people who take it in moderation. Because of that, it is widely considered to be safer than most prescription sedatives. However, there is always a very, very small risk that you will react to the herb in such a way that you cannot drive or operate heavy machinery. The chance of this happening is extremely small, but it still deserves mention. So it is generally best to try a test dose first at a time when you are relaxing (or trying to) at home.

To set your mind at ease, consider that a 1993 study of 40 subjects receiving kava extract determined that the herb had absolutely no effect on the participants' driving performance or their ability to operate heavy machinery. Kava calms and relaxes, but it does not fog the brain or impair judgement. The vast majority of users are able to do everything they could before—they just feel better while doing it.

"A lot of people think that kava will affect their thought processes like alcohol, marijuana, or prescription sedatives, but it doesn't work that way," says Sara, a 47-year-old freelance writer and longtime kava advocate. "For me, it has more of a calming effect than anything else. I drink a cup or two of kava tea after a hard day, and I feel pleasantly mellow. But kava doesn't knock me out; I still think clearly and my senses remain sharp. I just feel more relaxed and less stressed."

## Is it okay to supplement prescription medications with kava? I'm on a low-dose sedative for occasional anxiety problems, and I thought kava might enhance the effects of the medication.

It's never wise to mix drugs, and that goes for kava, too. Although it is a natural herb, kava still has pharmacologic effects, and for this reason, you should consult with your doctor before combining kava and sedatives, or any other medication.

This is especially true if you are on a benzodiazepine. An article in a recent issue of the *Annals of Internal Medicine* discussed the case of a patient who had to be hospitalized for disorientation and lethargy as a result of mixing Xanax (alprazolam) and kava. This incident suggests that kava can increase the sedative effect of benzodiazepines, which can be quite dangerous. As a result, people taking benzodiazepines should first consult their doctor and with the doctor's guidance be gradually weaned from the benzodiazepine before taking another medication, including kava. See Chapter 6: Side Effects for information on other potential side effects from kava.

## You've talked a lot about the effects of kava in easing stress and anxiety. What other medical problems can kava be used for?

Stress and anxiety are the two problems most commonly and widely treated with kava, but the herb has a wide array of other potential therapeutic uses. The natives of the South Pacific islands have used kava for centuries to treat a number of common conditions and there is anecdotal evidence that it can be effective, but few clinical studies on problems other than stress and anxiety have been performed. The handful of studies that have been conducted, however, have shown that kava may be generally useful.

A 1990 study on mice conducted by D. D. Jamieson and P. H. Duffield, for example, demonstrated that many of the active ingredients in kava—including kawain, dihydro-kawain, and methysticin—were effective in relieving mild pain. The physiology of this analgesic effect remains a mystery, although researchers are fairly sure that kava does not affect the brain the same way traditional opiate painkillers like morphine do. Anecdotal uses for kava as an analgesic and muscle relaxant include headaches, tooth-aches, menstrual cramps, and chronic neck pain, although the effect of kava is different from and nowhere near as strong as prescription analgesics. It can, however, reduce pain-related muscle tension, stress, and anxiety and thus make a painful condition easier to bear.

The muscle relaxant properties of kava have shown some promise in certain common female problems such as premenstrual syndrome (PMS) and recurrent urinary tract infections. No clinical studies have been conducted regarding kava and PMS, but anecdotal evidence from the Pacific islands suggests it can be beneficial in easing or eliminating many of the syndrome's most troublesome symptoms including anxiety, tension, irritability, and mood swings.

A little more is known about the effects of kava on the discomfort associated with urinary tract infections (UTIs). The herb's anesthetic properties, for example, make it useful in easing the painful burning sensation often felt in the urethra when UTIs are at their worst. Researchers at the University of Seattle in Washington have also found that kava can be effective in easing the pain of bladder infections by numbing the lining of the bladder. However, kava is not an antibiotic so it has no effect on a urinary tract infection itself. Traditional antibiotics are still required to eliminate the infection.

Studies at the University of Ulm in Germany also suggest that components in kava may one day make an effective blood thinner. Blood platelets tend to stick together, especially when exposed to a fatty acid known as arachidonic acid, and this can cause clots and other problems, particularly in heart and stroke patients. But in a 1997 study by Dr. J. Gleitz and colleagues, kawain inhibited the clumping of blood platelets exposed to arachidonic acid. This was a very preliminary study and the true strength of kava's anti-clotting properties has yet to be determined. Still, it suggests the wide potential benefits of certain herbal therapies and underscores the need for further research.

Kava also shows potential as an anti-inflammatory agent. In another study by Dr. Gleitz it was found that components of kava can inhibit the action of enzymes known as cyclooxygenase and thromboxane, thus preventing the formation of inflammation-causing chemicals prostaglandin $E_2$ and thromboxane $A_2$. A number of commercial non-steroidal anti-inflammatory drugs, such as ibuprofen, work in a similar fashion, so this finding is potentially significant. Kava has traditionally been used among the South Pacific islanders to ease inflammation in painful conditions such as arthritis, but many clinical studies will have to be performed before you can expect to see kava touted on store shelves as a safe and effective anti-inflammatory compound.

Even certain gastrointestinal conditions may benefit from regular doses of kava. In a 1997 study reported in the journal *Planta Medica*, kawain was found to relax certain smooth muscle cells in the small intestine of guinea pigs. If future studies find a similar reaction in humans, kava could one day be used to treat gastrointestinal problems stemming from an overactive small intestine, such as irritable bowel syndrome, which can be a symptom of anxiety. Not surprisingly, the South Pacific islanders have used kava to alleviate stomach and intestinal distress for hundreds of years.

**I've been under a lot of stress lately, and my doctor suggested I supplement my daily kava with melatonin. I thought melatonin was just to help people sleep. Can melatonin also help reduce the effects of stress and anxiety?**

Melatonin (which we will discuss at greater length in Chapter 5) is known primarily as a sleep aid, but studies have also found the hormone may be effective in curbing many of the ravages of daily stress.

Some doctors believe that stressed older people may benefit even more from melatonin than younger people because corticosteroids (a class of hormones that can spike dramatically during times of stress, as noted in Chapter 2: Stress and Anxiety) can remain at higher levels in their systems for longer periods of time, wreaking even greater havoc on already declining organs and systems.

Several studies have confirmed the beneficial effects of melatonin on an aging immune system. In one eye-opening 1995 study reported in the *Archives of Virology*, young and old mice were injected with an often fatal encephalitis virus. Half of each group was then given a daily dose of melatonin. Of the group that did not receive the hormone, only 6 percent of the young mice survived the virus and none of the older mice lived. But of the subjects that did receive melatonin, 39 percent of the young mice survived as did 56 percent of the older mice. While these results are very interesting, it must be remembered that the study was conducted on animals and clinical studies are needed to evaluate these finding in humans.

Melatonin is available in both tablet and capsule form and can be found at most grocery and health food stores. The proper daily dose depends on a number of factors, including age. Generally speaking, the older you are, the more melatonin you may need to achieve a therapeutic effect. The suggested dose for men and women in middle age (40 years and older) is around 1 milligram. Seniors (ages 55 and older) may start at 2 milligrams. Those 75 and older may require 3 milligrams or more, depending on their health. Because melatonin promotes sleep, it is most effective when taken at bedtime.

**A good friend of mine has started taking valerian for stress and anxiety, with good results. She says the herb is as effective as kava in relaxing her and helping her cope with the pressures of her job, which are numerous. Is valerian really an effective alternative to kava? Could you discuss this herb and whether or not it really works?**

Valerian has a long history as a therapeutic herb. It is commonly found throughout North America, Europe, and Asia and has been used medicinally since the time of ancient Greece. It was commonly used in the Middle Ages to treat gastrointestinal problems resulting from nervous tension and related ailments and later became revered as an effective relaxant and sleep aid. In fact, valerian was commonly used during World War I to ease the effects of shell shock. It remained in popular use in both Europe and the United States until the 1950s, when it was gradually replaced by chemical anxiolytics such as barbiturates and, later, benzodiazepines. However, valerian, as you have discovered, is starting to gain in popularity again as more and more people turn to herbal therapies.

The active ingredients in valerian are found primarily in the root. They include volatile oils such as valerenic acid and valenol, valepotriates, and alkaloids. Of all these compounds, the most potent, say herbalists, are the valepotriates. However, the plant contains literally dozens of chemical compounds and many of them have not been thoroughly documented or studied.

Valerian can be very effective, but researchers are still unsure exactly how it affects the body to reduce stress, induce a feeling of relaxation, and promote sleep. One theory, which has been supported by preliminary studies, suggests that it influences the same brain receptors as certain benzodiazepines. However, researchers are studying a variety of other possible mechanisms as well.

## Is valerian as potent as commercial sedatives?

No. Most prescription and over-the-counter sedatives and sleep aids—or hypnotics—are much stronger than valerian. For example, a 1993 German study in mice compared the sedative effect of valerian to diazepam (Valium) and chlorpromazine (Thorazine) and found valerian to be far less powerful. But most chemical sedatives and tranquilizers also can cause a significant number of side effects, which makes valerian a better choice in the eyes of many people.

Interestingly, a growing number of doctors are placing anxiety patients on valerian before trying more conventional drug therapies in the hope that the herb will be effective. Very often it is, although valerian, like any treatment, is not for everyone and reactions to the herb can vary widely. Valerian is widely considered to be extremely safe when consumed in recommended doses, but potential side effects can include stomach upset, restlessness, headaches, and even restless legs syndrome in a small number of users.

## In what forms is valerian available?

Valerian can be purchased at most health food stores in capsule, pill, liquid, and tea form. It is available in a number of different concentrations and combinations with other herbs, such as kava, hops, chamomile, or skullcap. As with any herb, it is best to start with a small dose and gradually increase it until you experience a reduction in anxiety symptoms. For mild anxiety, a single morning valerian dose of 150 to 300 milligrams is recommended, in addition to a 300 to 500 milligram dose one to two hours before bedtime. A concentrated root extract containing 0.5 to 1.0 percent of essential oils is a good start. If nothing happens, gradually increase the amount. Take your first dose on a day when you do not have to go to work or do anything important, just in case it makes you too drowsy to drive or perform other tasks that require significant alertness and concentration. Uncommonly, some people may experience morning sleepiness. If this is the case, reducing the dose should solve the problem. To maximize the potential for success, eliminate other dietary factors which can disrupt sleep, such as caffeine and alcohol. And remember: Consult your doctor first if you are on any kind of medication or suffer from any type of chronic illness. Valerian probably will not cause any problems, but it is always best to be safe. Researchers know little about the interaction of valerian and other common sedatives including alcohol, benzodiazepines, and barbiturates.

## Is it possible to overdose on valerian?

Yes, but even massive amounts of the herb appear to cause little toxicity. Dr. Leanna Willey and colleagues at the University of Rochester School of Medicine in Rochester, New York, reported in 1995 the story of an 18-year-old college student who tried to commit suicide by swallowing nearly 50 capsules containing 470 milligrams each of concentrated valerian root. Shortly after taking the capsules, the student experienced abdominal cramps, tightness in her chest, tremors in her extremities, and lightheadedness. She was rushed to the emergency room, where tests showed her vital signs and her heart, blood chemistry, and liver function all to be normal. She was given activated charcoal to absorb the valerian in her stomach (standard procedure in poison cases) and was fine the next day.

This incident suggests that valerian is safe even in very high doses, but it's unwise and potentially dangerous to intentionally push the envelope. No herb should ever be taken in extreme amounts because serious health problems could result in sensitive individuals. The girl described above was very lucky. Another person in a similar situation might not be.

**Is it okay for pregnant women to take valerian? I'd like to give it a try to ease my "new mom jitters" and help me sleep, but I don't want to do anything to endanger my baby.**

There have been no clinical studies on the effects of valerian on pregnant women or their babies. As with any prescription or over-the-counter medication or dietary supplement, pregnant or breast-feeding women should first consult their doctor before using herbs.

**Can valerian be addictive?**

There is little clinical or anecdotal evidence that valerian is addictive in healthy individuals who take it in recommended doses. However, it is possible that a user could become psychologically dependent on the herb to ease anxiety or induce sleep. For this reason it is a good idea to use valerian only when needed, rather than every day.

**I appreciate the information on kava and valerian. Are there any other herbs that can help relieve the symptoms of stress and anxiety? I feel much more comfortable turning to something natural rather than synthetic to ease these occasional problems.**

The herbal pharmacopoeia is full of medicinal herbs renowned for their ability to ease stress and anxiety; relax mind, body, and spirit; and help promote sleep (something we'll discuss at much greater length in the following chapter).

Indeed, herbs have been used for centuries around the world to calm jittery nerves and reduce stress. Some of the most widely recognized, aside from valerian, include passionflower, skullcap, hops, lemon balm, and chamomile.

Passionflower is an herbal anxiolytic with a long history of use. Indigenous to tropical areas of North America, it has been used for centuries to treat stress, anxiety, and certain kinds of pain.

Passionflower has a number of active ingredients, although the ones most useful to us are flavonoids such as isovitexin, orientin, kampferol, and vitexin, and indole alkaloids such as harmalin and harmol. These words mean little unless you are a botanist, but without them passionflower would be just another pretty plant.

There is quite a bit of anecdotal evidence regarding the effectiveness of passionflower in easing stress and anxiety and promoting sleep, but a 1997 study involving mice clearly demonstrated its sedative properties. When the mice received passionflower extract, they exhibited noticeably less anxious behavior, less activity, and fell into a state of drowsiness. Most people consume passionflower as a tea, although the herb is also available in capsule and tincture form. Like many other sleep-promoting herbs, it is most effective when taken shortly before bedtime.

As for side effects, passionflower has proved to be extremely safe when consumed in moderate quantities (one or two cups of tea, for example, or one or two capsules per evening). However, excessive amounts of passionflower could lead to heavy sedation and even affect consciousness, especially when combined with other herbs or commercial sedatives or anxiolytics. For this reason, it is wise to check with your doctor if you are on any type of medication or suffer from any type of chronic illness before using passionflower.

Skullcap, a member of the mint family indigenous to North America, is yet another herb that has been used for centuries to ease the effects of stress and anxiety in daily life. It can be used by itself or in combination with other calming herbs, especially chamomile. Despite a long history as an herbal therapeutic, researchers just a few short decades ago claimed skullcap to be useless. However, more recent research has uncovered a number of active ingredients in the plant, including volatile oils and flavonoids, that appear to induce mild sedation and to ease stress and anxiety and induce sleep. There is also anecdotal evidence that skullcap has antiviral and anti-inflammatory properties and can also ease the symptoms of premenstrual syndrome, although no clinical studies have confirmed this.

Skullcap is available in dried leaf, capsule, and tincture form, although it is most commonly found in premixed herbal combinations. Most people prefer the ease of capsules, but a cup of hot skullcap tea shortly before bedtime is a relaxing way to end the day. There are few side effects attributed to the normal consumption of skullcap; however, excessive doses can cause liver damage.

Chamomile has been used for centuries for a wide range of ailments. For example, the ancient Egyptians used it to treat malarial fever. In Europe the herb developed a reputation as a cure-all with reported mild sedative, anti-inflammatory, antispasmodic, and antibacterial properties. It reached the peak of its popularity to date in 1987 when the Germans named it the "plant of the year." While the sedative properties of chamomile have not been demonstrated in clinical studies, an abundance of anecdotal evidence has accumulated over the centuries supporting its calming effects.

Chamomile is most commonly used as a tea made from dried leaves or tincture, but some people prefer capsules because of their ease. Chamomile tea is readily available in most health food and grocery stores, but you may have to seek out an herbal specialty store for liquid tincture.

The active ingredients in chamomile include flavonoids such as chrysoplenin and apigenin, essential oils, and bisabolol. These compounds also aid digestion by relaxing the smooth muscles throughout the gastrointestinal system. Such effects were noted more than a century ago by Beatrix Potter in her tales of Peter Rabbit: "I am sorry to say that Peter was not very well during the evening. His mother put him to bed and made some chamomile tea; and she gave a dose to Peter! One tablespoon to be taken at bedtime." For best results, consume a cup of hot chamomile tea, or take one or two capsules after a heavy meal or shortly before bedtime. Side effects are rare, but sensitive individuals may experience an allergic reaction to chamomile. Discontinue use if allergy symptoms develop.

Many people who have tried the herbs discussed above swear by their stress-reducing abilities. "My doctor placed me on Valium for work-related anxiety, but I didn't like the side effects," says Karl, a 44-year-old corporate vice president. "I asked him for something a bit more natural, and he suggested chamomile and valerian. I was skeptical at first— how effective could plants be at easing anxiety and stress?—but they really worked. I've been using valerian as needed for several years with wonderful results. I also drink chamomile tea to help me sleep and to settle my stomach. Thanks to these and a number of other herbs, I'm no longer plagued by the symptoms of stress and anxiety. I actually look forward to getting up in the morning."

### I've read a lot about the use of St. John's Wort as a treatment for depression. Is there any indication that it can help relieve stress and anxiety?

St. John's Wort, known scientifically as *Hypericum perforatum*, has received quite a bit of publicity in recent months as an effective treatment for mild to moderate depression and other disorders. But it also has a long history—more than 2,000 years—as a folk remedy for nervousness, anxiety, and sleep problems. The clinical and anecdotal evidence for the use of St. John's Wort is so compelling that Germany's Commission E has approved the herb as a nonprescription remedy for anxiety, insomnia, and related ailments.

We believe St. John's Wort works by enhancing the effects of three essential neurotransmitters in the brain: dopamine, serotonin, and norepinephrine, although other neurotransmitters may also be involved. There is also some scientific evidence that the herb's active ingredients lower levels of cortisol, a hormone released during times of stress, and boost the effects of a natural brain neurotransmitter known as gamma-aminobutyric acid (GABA).

The amount of St. John's Wort necessary to reduce stress and anxiety differs from person to person and is predicated on a number of factors. As mentioned earlier, it is best to start with a small dose and gradually increase it until the desired effect is achieved. Most herbalists suggest starting with a daily dose of 300 milligrams three times a day. Studies have found this to be the optimum dose for most people, although you may need a little more or a little less depending on your health and degree of stress and anxiety.

St. John's Wort is widely recognized as safe, but there may be some minor side effects, including stomach upset or nausea. If this occurs, try taking the capsules with your meals. There is also a small risk of phototoxicity (sensitivity to sunlight) from taking St. John's Wort, so a sunscreen should be used if you spend a good deal of time outdoors. And if you are taking prescription antidepressant medication or any other kind of medication or suffer from a chronic illness, consult your doctor before starting St. John's Wort.

### Is St. John's Wort safe for pregnant women?

That's a good question. There has been very little clinical research on the use of St. John's Wort during pregnancy, although few problems have been reported after many years of use in Germany. Still, just to be safe, it is not wise to use St. John's Wort while pregnant or nursing unless your doctor says it is okay.

**Friends of mine have been taking very large doses of certain vitamins in the belief that megadoses can help them better cope with daily stress and anxiety. They have encouraged me to try a similar regimen, but I'm wary. Can megadoses of vitamins really help ease the symptoms of stress?**

Vitamins and minerals are essential nutrients, but there is very little scientific research to suggest that higher than recommended doses can help relieve stress. It is true that stress can adversely affect our diet and thus the amounts of essential nutrients we consume, but a generic multivitamin tablet can usually make up for any stress-related nutritional deficits.

In addition, health officials note that excessive amounts of certain vitamins and minerals can actually be unhealthy. Too much of one kind of nutrient can adversely affect the body's ability to absorb or use another. For example, taking more than 1,000 milligrams of vitamin C daily can decrease the availability of copper and selenium, causing a domino effect of poor nutrition. And certain nutrients, such as vitamins A and E, can actually be toxic in megadoses.

Don't listen to your friends; they are endangering their health with their excessive vitamin intake. There are far better and equally natural ways to keep stress and anxiety in check. Kava is just one of them.

**Speaking of diet, is it true that when we eat and how we combine our foods are just as important as what we eat when it comes to controlling the effects of stress?**

Yes. A balanced diet is extremely important in keeping your mind and body healthy and inhibiting the effects of daily stress, but nutrition experts say timing and amount can also play a role. For example, rather than eating the traditional three large meals a day, some people find that they benefit more from eating three smaller meals a day plus one or two snacks made up of complex carbohydrates such as bagels, fruit, or low-fat yogurt. This strategy helps fight stress by maintaining consistent blood sugar levels. It also helps prevent stress-induced indigestion, which can result from consuming a heavy meal on an upset stomach.

**My doctor recently suggested something called cognitive therapy to help relieve the effects of my anxiety. What is cognitive therapy and how does it work?**

To begin with, our thoughts are very closely tied to how we feel, both emotionally and physically. If you get praise from your boss or attention from an admirer, you may feel pretty good. On the other hand, if you fail a test despite hours of preparation or are passed up on that job promotion you had been counting on, you may feel sad and dejected. In fact, if other unpleasant things happen, you may start to think pretty negatively in general, feeling further depressed and hopeless. Cognitive therapy is a style of treatment, or psychotherapy, that many people find effective in breaking this cycle of negative thinking, which is a problem that afflicts many people with anxiety disorders. In a nutshell, it helps you to recognize the source of your trouble and replace fear-provoking thoughts with positive encouragment.

One of the most effective forms of cognitive therapy is known as self-talk, and it works just as the name suggests. Whenever you start to feel overwhelmed by anxiety-producing thoughts or sensations, repeat either aloud or to yourself instructions to disregard such negative thinking. For example, if you find yourself worrying about work to the point where you are overcome by anxiety, repeat to yourself: "This problem is no worse than any other. I can get the job done. There's no need to worry." Do this every time stress or anxiety raise their ugly heads and pretty soon you will find your anxiety-related symptoms becoming increasingly less common. In fact, you may be able to get rid of them completely. Many anxiety patients find it helpful to write down the positive thoughts that most effectively replace negative thinking and keep that list with them at all times. Your doctor may be able to recommend other forms of cognitive therapy more appropriate for your specific condition.

# FIVE

⟨━━━⟩

## *Treating Insomnia with Kava and Other Remedies*

*FACT:* Kava has been used as a natural sleep aid by the people of the South Pacific islands for hundreds, perhaps thousands of years, and is widely prescribed throughout Europe.

*FACT:* Studies have shown that kava promotes and supports the natural cycles of sleep much more effectively than most prescription medications—and with minimal side effects.

*FACT:* There are very few anecdotal reports of "kava hangover." In fact, most kava users say the herb leaves them feeling great the next morning.

*FACT:* Kava can be useful in reducing the amount of a prescription medication needed to induce sleep.

*FACT:* A cure for insomnia doesn't have to break your wallet. Other inexpensive natural sleep aids include valerian, hops, California poppy, and the hormone melatonin.

⟨━━━⟩

*Insomnia had become a way of life for Sandra. The 38-year-old kindergarten teacher thought at first that her inability to fall asleep was a temporary problem that would correct itself in a day or so. But the days dragged into weeks and the weeks into months until Sandra came to view her sleep disruption as just another indication that she was growing older.*

After the first week of sleeplessness Sandra tried a popular over-the-counter sleep aid but woke up feeling groggy and out of sorts. She later mentioned the problem to her doctor during her annual check-up, and she was given a prescription for a medication that was supposed to help her sleep. But Sandra threw the pills away after one try because they left her so groggy that she slept through her alarm clock and was two hours late for work.

"I stopped trying after that," Sandra confesses. "I was tired all the time because no matter when I went to bed, my mind wouldn't stop racing and it would be hours before I finally fell asleep. And even then, I slept fitfully. I never felt really rested, even on weekends, but I came to believe that my problem was simply part of today's hectic lifestyle. Half of my girlfriends complained of insomnia, and after a few months I just grew to accept it. I didn't like it, but there didn't seem to be much I could do about it."

Then Sandra was introduced to kava. While visiting an aunt in another state, Sandra happened to mention her inability to get a good night's sleep, even on vacation. "I told her about my bad experiences with sleep medications, and she asked if I had tried any herbal remedies," Sandra recalls. "I said I hadn't, and she pulled out a bottle of kava tablets. 'Try these,' she said. 'They really help me when I'm stressed and can't sleep.'"

Sandra admits to being skeptical about the herb, but she figured that she had nothing to lose. On her aunt's recommendation, she took two tablets after dinner. Within an hour, she started to feel relaxed and mellow. "It was like a minor alcohol buzz without the impaired thinking," Sandra notes. "It was very pleasant. My aunt and I had a wonderful chat, and around 11 PM I started to feel really drowsy. I went to *bed and slept all the way through for the first time in recent memory."*

*Not surprisingly, Sandra is now a vocal advocate of kava. She started taking it nightly after she returned from vacation, then gradually cut back as her sleep pattern returned to normal. "I still take it after a particularly stress-ful day, but it's not something I'm dependent on," Sandra says. "I usually sleep pretty well now, but on those evenings when I feel overly restless or anxious, it helps calm my nerves and promotes drowsiness. Best of all, I wake up feel-ing great. There's no sleeping-pill hangover!"*

Sandra is one of a growing number of Americans who have said no to prescription sleep medications and yes to kava. The herb is known primarily for its stress and anxiety-busting properties, but centuries of use in the South Pacific islands have also proved its usefulness in combating insom-nia and other sleep disorders and restoring normal sleep pat-terns. Best of all, it works with no side effects when taken in recommended doses.

In this chapter we will discuss the use of kava in easing insomnia, the forms in which it is most useful, and the many other herbal hypnotics currently on the market.

**I know that kava has a long history as a medicinal herb and that it is widely touted as an effective sleep aid. But is there any substantial clinical research to back up this claim?**

Yes, although not nearly the amount of research verify-ing kava's effectiveness as a treatment for stress and anxi-ety. Most of the evidence regarding kava's sleep-inducing properties is anecdotal—but there's a lot of it!

In one well-regarded study conducted by Dr. W. Emser and colleagues at Ceritas Hospital in Dillingen, Germany, 12 subjects between the ages of 20 and 31 were divided into two groups, with each group receiving a 50 milligram or a

100 milligram dose of standardized kava extract three times a day. Physiological responses were monitored over the experiment's four days and nights using an electroencephalograph (EEG), an electromyograph (EMG), and other devices.

The results of this study were intriguing. For example, sleep-spindle density (bursts of activity during early sleep, as seen on EEG) was about 20 percent higher in 11 of the 12 subjects receiving kava regardless of dose, suggesting that the herb enhances sleep function much like prescription sedatives, but without the side effects or deep-sleep suppression. In addition, it was found that deep and slow-wave sleep—stages 3 and 4, as discussed in Chapter 3—was increased without any noticeable changes in the rapid-eye-movement (REM) phase. And subjects reported no REM rebound when they stopped taking kava.

What does all of this mean? That kava induces and supports the natural cycles of sleep much more effectively than most prescription medications—something users have known for a long time.

## How does kava help us sleep?

Researchers are still trying to figure out the specific action that makes kava such a terrific sleep aid for many people, although obviously its ability to induce a state of muscular relaxation plays an important role, as evidenced by a 1962 study on mice conducted by researcher H. J. Meyer. Later animal studies by Meyer and others also linked the administration of specific kavalactones, primarily dihydromethysicin and dihydrokawain, to the sedation and onset of sleep typically seen in kava use, although again the specific action has yet to be fully explained. Pigeons given the herb slept for up to 10 hours, and monkeys slept for up to 15 hours.

There is no doubt that kava induces a state of drowsiness in the majority of people who take it. But more research is needed to understand exactly how it works.

## Is kava an effective sleep aid for everyone? Do all users derive the same benefits?

No. Sleep trouble is a very common feature of many, many conditions, such as depression or anxiety. In many cases identifying and treating the cause of the sleep disturbance generally solves the problem, although a short course of kava may also be helpful. In other cases, however, sleep disruption may be related to our responses to the hassles of day-to-day life or, less commonly, to a sleep disorder called primary insomnia. Kava may be very effective for these types of insomia as well.

Remember that, as with anything, people react differently when using kava. Anecdotal research has shown that some users quickly become quite drowsy as a result of consuming kava, while others find that the herb mellows them out but does not induce drowsiness at all. The most commonly reported effect, however, is an initial burst of alertness, followed a few hours later by drowsiness.

A number of factors can play a significant role in how kava affects you as a sleep aid including when you consume it, how you consume it, the quality of the kava you are using, the size of the dose, and your overall health. Practicing good sleep hygiene will also help you to get the full benefit from kava. Before you go to bed, avoid caffeine, alcohol, and that late-night snack. And if you exercise, do so at least three hours before you plan to retire.

## I suffer from occasional bouts of sleeplessness and kava sounds like something that could really help. When should I take kava for maximum effectiveness?

Most herbalists suggest taking kava at least a couple of hours before you plan to go to bed. If you take it right at bedtime, you may become more alert at first, and that could keep you awake longer than you want to be.

## How much kava should I take to help me sleep at night?

That depends on a number of factors, including the potency of the kava you are taking and your own system. Some types of kava are more sedating than others, although there's really no way to determine that with most commercial products. Also, people react differently to kava. Some fall asleep quickly on a small dose, while others require much more.

Most people learn what works best for them through trial and error, but one to two capsules containing 60 or 70 milligrams of kavalactones each is a good starting dose. If you do not feel drowsy after a few hours, gradually increase the dose over a couple of days until you achieve the desired effect. Some people need more than 140 milligrams of kavalactones to experience the benefits of kava. However, higher doses are safe, but should not exceed 500 to 800 milligrams kavalactones and should be used for short term use only.

The majority of users find that kava capsules work quite well, although some say they get their best sleep after drinking a couple of cups of kava tea made from dried root or tincture, possibly because it is an integral part of their bedtime ritual. The choice is yours—if one form doesn't work for you, try the other.

## Can kava leave you feeling woozy or groggy the morning after you use it like certain prescription medications do?

There are very few anecdotal reports of "kava hangover." In fact, most kava aficionados say the herb leaves them feeling great the next morning. This effect is often caused by the deep sleep that can accompany kava use. Studies have shown that kava, unlike many prescription medications, does not interfere with the many stages we go through during a night of sound sleep, so we wake up feeling rested and relaxed. Prescription sedatives knock us out, but they don't promote healthy sleep, which really makes their use a catch-22.

### Is it okay to combine kava with a prescription sedative? I'm on a prescription hypnotic to help me sleep, and I was hoping that kava could make it work even better.

You should combine drugs (and in this case kava counts as a drug, albeit a natural, less hazardous one) *only* under the supervision of your doctor. Kava may potentiate, or make more active, the effects of many prescription sleep aids, so there is a serious risk of oversedation if you take too much kava on top of your other medication.

However, there is a potential good side to this effect in that kava could be useful in reducing the amount of a prescription medication needed to induce sleep. In fact, over a period of time, kava could in certain cases help eliminate the need for prescription medications altogether. But such a program should not be attempted on your own. Talk to your doctor and ask for help in weaning you from prescription sedatives and on to kava.

### My husband is very restless in bed at night, and since we sleep in the same bed, it affects me, too. His legs jerk violently all night long, which means I don't get a lot of sleep. I'm ready to move into a separate bedroom! Could kava be helpful in alleviating this condition?

It sounds like your husband has a condition known as periodic limb movement disorder (PLM). This condition is characterized by repetitive, unvarying limb movements that occur in sleep. It may occur only occasionally or dozens, even hundreds of times a night. Another common condition which may affect sleep is restless legs syndrome (RLS). Restless legs syndrome is characterized by disagreeable leg sensations that usually occur prior to falling asleep and can cause an irresistible urge to move the legs. Whatever the cause of your husband's affliction, as you have found out, it can be a problem for both bed partners—and some couples have even gotten divorced over it.

But periodic limb movement disorder and restless legs syndrome can be more than a simple irritation. In extreme cases, these disorders can interfere with sleep to such a degree that all concerned are constantly exhausted. After a while, people suffering from either of these disorders may find that their immune systems may start to weaken so they get sick more often, mental processes such as memory and concentration begin to deteriorate, they become irritable, and their stress levels go through the roof. The result: Both their work and home lives suffer greatly.

There are a few prescription medications for the control of periodic limb movement disorder and restless legs syndrome (see Chapter 3: Insomnia for more information), but kava may also prove helpful by promoting muscular relaxation as well as a deep, restful sleep. There is more anecdotal evidence than clinical research regarding this use of kava, but it is definitely worth a try. If it does not work, your doctor may be able to suggest some more effective alternatives.

**I think I have chronic fatigue syndrome and it's making my life a living hell. I'm tired all the time and I have almost no energy at all. My doctor treats me symptomatically but has yet to find a specific medical explanation for my condition. Even though I'm constantly fatigued, I don't sleep well at night, which only makes my physical problems worse. Could kava help?**

The symptoms you describe—constant tiredness, lack of energy, poor sleep—are common features of a variety of conditions. For example, these symptoms are very frequently reported by people who are depressed and/or have generalized anxiety. In these cases, treating the depression or the anxiety usually solves the problem. Less commonly, however, these symptoms may be attributable to chronic fatigue syndrome. If other conditions have been ruled out by your doctor, you may indeed have chronic fatigue syndrome.

Chronic fatigue syndrome has been the source of much debate within the medical community for a number of years. Some researchers believe it is a specific disease, possibly autoimmune or viral in origin, while others are not so sure. A lot of research is being conducted on chronic fatigue syndrome (which goes by a number of names), but at the moment there are more questions than answers.

The one thing that is known is that this is an agonizing condition that can wreak havoc on the lives of its victims and their families. Common symptoms include headache, low-grade fever, swelling of the lymph nodes, muscle and joint pain, and intestinal problems. Sleep deprivation is a secondary complaint afflicting many people with this condition, and it is here that kava may be most useful. Although it is certainly not a cure for chronic fatigue syndrome, kava may be able to ease accompanying anxiety and help sufferers get a good night's sleep. This in turn may strengthen their weakened immune systems and enable them to cope a little better with some of the disorder's more bothersome symptoms.

Kava also has a reputation as an analgesic, and regular use of the herb may help ease some of the more painful symptoms commonly associated with chronic fatigue syndrome such as sore throat and headache. However, the severity of the condition may necessitate stronger measures.

If your doctor has you on a prescription medication for your condition, make sure that you mention that you are also taking kava.

**My husband, after years of excessive drinking, has
finally realized that he's an alcoholic and has
joined Alcoholics Anonymous. It's a rough road,
but he's confident he can beat his drinking problem and I'm helping him every way I can. Before he
sought help, my husband would often go to bed
drunk and sleep fitfully. I thought that once he
stopped drinking, his sleep would improve, but
that doesn't seem to be happening. He's also experiencing some other physical problems as his body
goes through withdrawal. Could kava help him
sleep better and aid his quest to stay sober?**

Kicking an addictive substance like alcohol is never
easy, and most alcoholics find the first few weeks of their
recovery extremely difficult as their bodies go through the
process of cleansing themselves. Long-term alcoholics may
suffer symptoms of physical withdrawal during the first few
days of detoxification that can include nausea, fever, muscle spasms, trembling, sweating, diarrhea, and in more
severe cases, hallucinations and even seizures. Sleep disruption is also a common complaint during recovery and
can last for several weeks.

Many doctors prescribe low doses of anxiety-easing
medications, usually benzodiazepines, for people going
through alcohol withdrawal to help ease some of the symptoms. These medications are usually prescribed as a brief
taper to be discontinued after a week or so. In rare cases, the
individual may stay on the benzodiazepine for a longer
period, a situation that raises the concern that the individual
will develop an addiction of another kind. In cases where
this is a potential risk, or if a more natural approach to long-
term recovery is preferred, kava may be an effective alternative or adjunct for a number of reasons. Kava can help to
ease the discomfort experienced in the immediate withdrawal period. Kava may also reduce the underlying anxiety that is commonly seen in alcoholics; many people who

feel anxious start drinking to calm themselves and after years of drinking, the situation ultimately gets out of hand. However, if you have had significant withdrawal symptoms when discontinuing drinking in the past (such as hallucinations, seizures, or delirium tremors), you should seek a doctor's assistance with your detoxification.

To evaluate the effectiveness of kava during alcohol withdrawal, Dr. K. Kryspin-Exner, a psychiatrist at the University of Vienna in Austria, gathered 50 recovering alcoholics and divided them into two groups. One group received one 200 milligram capsule of the kavalactone kawain three times a day for five weeks, and the other group received a placebo. Before the start of the study, 28 of the subjects had been treated with a prescription sedative/hypnotic during the first three to five days of severe withdrawal, and all of the subjects were given a multivitamin by injection during the same time period.

The results of the study were better than expected: Twenty-three of the 25 subjects receiving kawain reported noticeably less fear, anxiety, fatigue, dizziness, loss of appetite, and other symptoms. By comparison, 11 of the 25 subjects receiving a placebo complained of withdrawal symptoms. Dr. Kryspin-Exner also found that the kawain was well tolerated by the subjects and—better still— showed no indication of being addictive. There was no mention in Dr. Kryspin-Exner's report on kava and sleep, but it is highly likely that those receiving kawain were able to sleep better than those on the placebo simply because their other withdrawal symptoms were less severe.

**Kava can be beneficial to a lot of people afflicted with insomnia, but as you noted earlier, it may not be for everyone. Could you discuss some of the other effective herbal sleep aids currently available in grocery and health food stores?**

Herbs were used to induce a good night's sleep long before any synthetic drugs were created, and there is a wealth of anecdotal evidence supporting their effectiveness. Indeed, nearly every ancient culture had its herbal medicine chest and it is interesting to note that our attitudes toward herbalism are starting to come full circle again as people realize the wisdom of our forefathers.

One of the best known herbal treatments for insomnia is valerian, which was discussed briefly in Chapter 4 as an herbal treatment for anxiety and stress. Valerian has a well-documented sedative effect and is widely used throughout Europe for the treatment of sleeplessness. But its use as a sleep aid actually goes back thousands of years to ancient India and China, where the plant was—and still is—a highly regarded part of traditional medicine.

A number of clinical studies have confirmed valerian's value as a sleep aid, including its ability to prevent nightmares and unwanted nighttime awakening. In several different studies the herb reduced the time it took test subjects to fall asleep and dramatically improved the quality of sleep, even among those who consumed a lot of coffee and other compounds with stimulating properties.

Other clinical studies have found that valerian promotes sleep as effectively as certain benzodiazepine sedatives, but without affecting memory or concentration. In a 1996 German study by U. Gerhard and colleagues, the effects of valerian were compared to a benzodiazepine, flurazepam (Dalmane), and a placebo in the treatment of insomnia. Nearly 50 percent of the 20 subjects receiving the benzodiazepine complained of side effects compared to only 10 percent of the valerian group. Both compounds worked equally well at easing sleeplessness.

Valerian is available in many forms and in many strengths. As a treatment for insomnia, most herbalists suggest a starting dose of 150 to 300 milligrams of standardized valerian containing 0.8 to 1.0 percent valerenic acid taken about an hour before you go to bed, with a gradual increase in dose until sleep comes easily. A tea made from dried root or tincture is also effective. However, you may not experience any benefits right away. It sometimes takes two weeks or more of regular use before the herb's sleep-inducing action really takes effect, which makes it less desirable for cases of chronic insomnia. But once valerian kicks in, it usually works well and with minimal side effects when consumed in recommended doses. After sleep patterns are normalized, the use of valerian can be tapered off.

As a side note, valerian may also benefit people who are hooked on prescription sleep medications by both helping them to kick the habit and acting as an effective substitute. In a 1994 study in rats, valerian very effectively helped reduce the symptoms of benzodiazepine withdrawal and there is strong evidence to suggest that it could work equally well on humans. However, consult your doctor before starting such a plan yourself. Withdrawal and substitution should be done very gradually because the sudden cessation of benzodiazepines, especially after long-term use, could cause dangerous side effects, including seizures.

"I tried valerian after several weeks of sleeplessness and found it very effective," notes Kelly, a 33-year-old book editor. "I tried a commercial valerian tea and it induced drowsiness about an hour or so after I drank it. Best of all, I slept very well throughout the night. I continued to rely on valerian for a couple of weeks, and then slowly cut down because I no longer seemed to need it. I still have a box of valerian tea bags in my kitchen, though, for those nights when I just can't seem to fall asleep. It's effective and it makes me feel good to know that it has no side effects. Quite frankly, that's the reason I never tried traditional sleep medications."

Also effective in the treatment of sleeplessness is hops, which is known primarily as an ingredient in beer. The plant is indigenous to North America, Asia, and Europe and has a long history as an herbal curative. Since ancient times, hops have been used as a tonic, diuretic, topical bactericidal, and digestive therapeutic, and later as a sleep aid. One of the first indications of hops' sedative effects was the fact that farm hands who picked the herb grew tired very easily, apparently as a result of ingesting hops resin into their bodies.

Hops has a number of active ingredients, including flavonoids, resins, and weak acids such as humulone, lupulin, and humulene. But researchers believe a chemical called dimethylvinyl carbinol is responsible for its ability to calm the system and induce sleep. A variety of products containing standardized hops, either alone or in combination with other tranquilizing herbs such as valerian, are available in grocery or health food stores. It can also be consumed in a tea made from dried flowers or tincture. A good starting dose is 500 milligrams of standardized dried hops in capsule or an equivalent extract-based product taken an hour or so before retiring. If the capsules do not bring on sleep quickly enough, gradually increase the dose until the desired effect is achieved. Most commercial hops products work well, promoting restful sleep without morning grogginess. Some companies also sell special pillows filled with hops, but the contents should be changed frequently because fresh hops lose their effectiveness rather quickly.

Hops is generally regarded as safe when consumed in recommended amounts, and there are few reports of side effects from taking the herb. However, because of its sedative effects, hops should not be taken in high doses by people who must drive an automobile or by those who are depressed as it may accentuate the depressive symptoms. Hops should also be avoided by those who are on prescription sedatives except under the supervision of a doctor.

Herbalists report that passionflower and chamomile, while not quite as effective as valerian or hops, can also help bring about a sense of calm and induce restful sleep in many people suffering from insomnia.

Passionflower has an extensive history as a sedative herb, but researchers have only recently verified its efficacy in laboratory studies. In one 1997 study, for example, mice who were given passionflower extract demonstrated less anxious behavior, a decrease in activity, and quickly grew drowsy. The water extract of passionflower was considerably more effective than the alcohol extract, suggesting that the best way to consume passionflower for better sleep is in tea form. The herb is also available as a capsule and tincture at most grocery and health food stores.

Very few side effects have been associated with passionflower when consumed in recommended doses. However, studies suggest that excessive amounts, especially if combined with other sedating herbs or prescription medications, could result in oversedation and even a change in consciousness. For best results, take one or two capsules of standardized passionflower or a cup of passionflower tea about an hour or so before bedtime. If sleep is slow in coming, gradually increase the dose as needed.

Although chamomile may not be as potent as other herbs, a couple of capsules or a cup of chamomile tea in the evening can be a pleasant way to relax and calm down after a tough day at the office. A second cup an hour or so before bedtime can help induce drowsiness even more. In addition, weak chamomile tea can be particularly helpful in soothing colicky or teething infants, and the herb is renowned throughout the world as an effective digestive aid. Strong anecdotal evidence suggests that chamomile is especially useful in calming gastrointestinal disorders caused by stress and anxiety, such as irritable bowel syndrome.

Chamomile is widely available in capsule, tincture, and tea form. But because the sedating effect of chamomile is much gentler than that of valerian, hops, or other plants, chamomile may prove ineffective for people suffering from more severe forms of insomnia. In such cases, chamomile should be used in combination with stronger herbs.

Chamomile is generally regarded as safe if consumed in recommended doses. However, there is a small risk of allergic reaction in sensitive people, especially those who have other allergies. As an extreme example, the *Journal of Allergy and Clinical Immunology* noted the case of an eight-year-old boy who experienced a near-fatal reaction to chamomile tea. Apparently the reaction was exacerbated by a long history of hay fever and bronchial asthma caused by a variety of common plant pollens. More mild reactions, such as itchy eyes, have also been reported after consuming chamomile tea. Discontinue use if allergy symptoms occur and try some of the other sedating herbs discussed above.

**An employee at my local health food store suggested California poppy to help me sleep on those occasional nights when insomnia is a problem. I had never heard of this plant before. Could it be useful?**

The California poppy has sleep-inducing as well as mild anxiolytic (anxiety-easing) properties. Although not quite as popular as valerian, hops, chamomile, and other sedating herbs, California poppy is quickly gaining a devoted following as more and more people eschew prescription medications in favor of a more natural approach to health care.

The California poppy is a distant relative of the opium poppy, but its active ingredients are far less potent and are nonaddictive. The herb is available in most health food stores in dried form and as a tincture, which has a very bitter taste. A few drops of tincture or a spoonful of powdered herb makes an effective tea, though the tincture may need to be sweetened with honey or mixed with fruit juice. For best results, drink the tea an hour or so before you plan to go to bed.

While it has not yet received approval from Germany's Commission E, an organization that approves the use of herbs for medicinal purposes, California poppy is considered generally safe and effective when consumed in recommended doses. Consult the accompanying literature for the proper dose.

## Can St. John's Wort be used to treat insomnia?

Yes, especially when sleeplessness is a result of mild to moderate depression. As discussed earlier, St. John's Wort—known botanically as hypericum—has a long history as an herbal antidepressant, and numerous clinical studies have confirmed this action. Insomnia in various forms often accompanies depression, so the daily use of St. John's Wort may be effective in reestablishing healthy sleep patterns.

It should be noted, however, that severe depression may require something stronger than St. John's Wort, which is a decision that should be made by your doctor. In most cases, depression-related insomnia improves when the depression starts to disappear.

## I've been hearing a lot about the effectiveness of melatonin in the treatment of insomnia. Does this compound really work, or is it just hype?

Melatonin is not just hype—researchers have confirmed without question the hormone's ability to induce a sound, restful sleep without disrupting the many important stages of sleep and with none of the side effects commonly associated with prescription medications. In fact, the National Aeronautics and Space Administration (NASA) is investigating the possible use of melatonin as a sleep aid for space shuttle astronauts.

In a study conducted at Brooks Air Force Base in San Antonio, Texas, volunteers reported to a sleep lab early one morning following a good night's sleep. All felt rested and restored. At 9 AM, the subjects were given a pill containing 10 milligrams of melatonin, 100 milligrams of melatonin, or a placebo. They were then free to play video games or occupy themselves however else they wished. Every two hours the subjects were given a battery of tests. At noon, one of the subjects who had received a 100 milligram dose of melatonin fell into a gentle sleep while playing a video game, proving the sleep-inducing abilities of the hormone even in people who are not otherwise fatigued.

Researchers note that melatonin also works well in much lower doses. Studies have shown that 10 milligrams or less of melatonin can bring about a sound sleep, especially in those who are exhausted or otherwise sleep deprived. In a 1995 study, volunteers were divided into two groups. One group received 1 milligram of melatonin and the other group received just 0.3 milligrams of the hormone. Both groups became drowsy and fell asleep in less time than usual.

Yet another study found melatonin just as effective as some benzodiazepines in promoting sleep. Test subjects, who were allowed to sleep in their own beds while hooked up to sleep monitors, were given either 10 milligrams of melatonin, the benzodiazepine temazepam (Restoril), or a placebo. Not surprisingly, those given melatonin fell asleep just as quickly as those receiving temazepam and slept for a similar length of time. But melatonin proved to be the better compound in that it did not delay REM sleep or affect the normal sleep cycle like the temazepam did.

Melatonin can work well for many people, but studies suggest it holds special promise for seniors, who often don't sleep well because of an age-related reduction in normal melatonin production and changes in the melatonin cycle. The most common complaint among people who are melatonin deficient is becoming drowsy too early in the evening and waking up too early in the morning. But a daily dose of melatonin can maintain healthy levels of the hormone and in turn can promote a more normal and restful sleep cycle. A standard dose for older people has yet to be determined, but 0.5 to 5 milligrams taken at night appears to work well for most. When adjusting your dosage, however, you should always remember the adage "start low, go slow." As a side note, melatonin can also help people whose melatonin production is out of phase because they work the swing shift or travel frequently.

Bottom line: Melatonin is an effective sleep aid with no known side effects. It promotes healthy sleep, does not interfere with sleep stages or patterns, and leaves users feeling rested and refreshed in the morning. Best of all, it's readily available in a variety of doses and very inexpensive compared to most prescription medications. A good starting dose is 0.5 to 3 milligrams taken about 30 minutes before bedtime. If you awaken in the middle of the night, gradually increase your dose until you sleep well throughout the night.

"Melatonin is wonderful for those nights when you just can't fall asleep," attests Kathy, a 23-year-old graphic artist. "It works quickly, induces a very restful sleep, and leaves you feeling great in the morning. Best of all, there are no side effects or bizarre interactions."

"I usually sleep pretty well, but sometimes I develop insomnia when I'm working on a difficult project and deadlines are weighing on me. My mind races during those times and I can't seem to calm myself down enough to fall asleep the way I should. When that happens, 5 milligrams of melatonin puts me out in no time. I also take it with me when I travel to help me fall asleep in unfamiliar surroundings."

## Melatonin sounds like a miracle compound! How does it help us fall asleep?

While there is no doubt that melatonin works, researchers are at odds over how it induces sleep so effectively. Some believe that the hormone, which is produced naturally by the pineal gland in the brain, affects our circadian cycle so that we fall asleep sooner. Others speculate that it has a more direct action, which has yet to be explained.

Studies show, however, that some definite physiological changes occur when you consume melatonin—pulse rate slows, temperature drops, reaction time slows, stress and tension melt away, and drowsiness increases. All of these combine to make sleep easier and more restful.

**I currently care for my father, who has mid-stage Alzheimer's disease. He doesn't sleep well and is up much of the night, which means I don't sleep much either. A member of my Alzheimer's disease support group suggested I give my father melatonin at bedtime to help him sleep longer. Will it work? Is it safe?**

Sleeplessness is one of the most frequently reported effects of Alzheimer's disease, and it is also one of the most common reasons people with the disorder are placed in long-term care facilities; their loved ones simply become too exhausted to care for them properly at home. But melatonin may help. In a study conducted at Oregon Health Sciences University, small amounts of melatonin given in a time-release pill at bedtime safely helped patients with Alzheimer's disease sleep as much as two hours longer. Interestingly, the researchers noted that those who responded the best were those who had the greatest difficulty sleeping.

Consult with your father's doctor about the use of melatonin in helping your father sleep a little better. And make sure that you do not become so exhausted in caring for your father that your own health suffers.

**Is there anyone who can't be helped with melatonin?**

Melatonin can be a godsend for many people afflicted with various types of insomnia, but it is not a cure-all. It probably won't be of much help to people who are kept awake by chronic pain, extreme anxiety, or serious depression. Such individuals generally need more help than melatonin alone can provide.

One possible answer is a combination of melatonin and other medications. Researchers at Oregon Health Sciences

University, for example, are looking into the effectiveness of a melatonin-benzodiazepine combination for people who cannot sleep because of anxiety-related problems. Preliminary findings suggest that such a combination can induce a more healthy sleep state than benzodiazepines alone, but additional studies are needed for confirmation.

**Occasionally I'll take kava too late in the evening and it keeps me awake when I'd rather be asleep. When that happens, is it safe to combine kava with other natural sleep-inducing compounds?**

Yes. Other sedative herbs such as valerian, chamomile, skullcap, and passionflower are safe and effective alternatives when kava makes you alert rather than putting you to sleep. A capsule or two, or a cup of herbal tea, can usually counter the stimulating effects of kava and help you to fall asleep in no time. The hormone melatonin can also be effective in doses of up to 5 milligrams taken about 30 minutes before you go to bed.

Remember, however, that kava very often has a sedating effect hours after that initial feeling of alertness, so you must be careful when combining it with other sleep-inducing compounds. Take too much and you could experience oversedation, which potentially could leave you feeling a bit out of sorts the next day. There have been no clinical studies on this issue, but the wise thing would be to consume half of a standard dose of other sedative herbs when taking them in combination with kava. The easiest solution for you, however, would be to take kava at least two hours before retiring to bed.

**A friend of mine is taking something called 5-HTP for sleep problems. It sounds like it's working, but my friend couldn't tell me what it is. Could you discuss this compound?**

Your friend is taking 5-hydroxytryptophan, more commonly known as 5-HTP. While this compound is available over-the-counter, 5-HTP is a naturally occurring substance we all possess and is a precursor to an important chemical, serotonin, which is found in the brain and gut. Some studies have suggested that it may have antidepressant effects. It can also help to induce a restful sleep. Most people have found that taking between 20 and 50 milligrams of 5-HTP an hour or so before bedtime helps them sleep deeply and well, with no side effects in the morning. 5-HTP can also be used to curb the stimulating effects of kava if the herb is consumed too close to bedtime.

### Can kava help travelers recover from the effects of jet lag?

There is some anecdotal evidence that suggests that kava can help induce sleep in people stricken with jet lag, but the herb apparently has little effect in helping the body reset its circadian rhythms. According to sleep experts, melatonin or 5-HTP would probably be more effective.

**My aunt suffered from occasional insomnia until she started playing around with aromatherapy. She burns incense in her bedroom and says it helps her calm down and sleep well. Can aromatherapy really help someone fall asleep? It all sounds too easy.**

Aromatherapy is becoming one of the hottest therapies of the 1990s, and with good reason—it often works. This is especially true of aromatherapy's use in the treatment of insomnia, a condition that reacts well to calming, soothing, sedating fragrances.

According to practitioners, aromatherapy helps normalize poor sleep patterns by relaxing the mind and body. The most effective essential oils for sleep are lavender, chamomile, sandalwood, frankincense, and clary sage. They can be applied in a number of ways, such as a fragrant massage oil, bath oil, or bedroom incense.

"I find that aromatherapy works best when used in conjunction with a calming bedtime ritual of soft music and low light," says Erin, a 48-year-old mother of three who has used essential oils to help her sleep for years. "The combination of soothing fragrances and mellow music makes me drowsy to the point where I'm asleep almost as soon as my head hits the pillow. It's effective, and a lot safer than prescription pills."

Aromatic essential oils and incense can be found in many health food and New Age stores.

## My grandmother used to give me a glass of warm milk when I had trouble sleeping as a child. Is this still a recommended treatment for insomnia?

No. Warm milk to induce sleep is actually an old wive's tale that has been disproved by clinical research.

Milk used to be the insomnia cure of choice because it contains an amino acid called tryptophan. In a number of studies, high levels of tryptophan were found to induce drowsiness, so it was assumed that milk and other tryptophan-rich foods like turkey would have a similar effect. But when researchers at the Massachusetts Institute of Technology (MIT) tried to confirm this, they found just the opposite to be true. Drinking milk is an ineffective insomnia cure because it actually causes tryptophan levels in the brain to fall as other amino acids from milk push the small amount of the chemical aside in their rush to get into the brain.

In fact, skim milk or low-fat milk can actually stimulate the brain rather than sedate it because of the presence of tyrosine, which triggers production of dopamine and norepinephrine—chemicals that tend to be more stimulating.

More beneficial in your quest for sleep are small amounts of carbohydrates such as honey, sugar, bread, potatoes, or rice, say MIT food researchers. It's an old wive's tale that sugar stimulates; current research has found that it actually sedates. In fact, many people find that an ounce or so of carbohydrate-rich foods at bedtime puts them to sleep faster than anything else without side effects or morning drowsiness. Researchers are unsure why, although it has been speculated that carbohydrates improve the transmission of serotonin and other sleep- and mood-affecting brain chemicals.

In addition, you should lay off alcohol and caffeine-rich coffee, tea, chocolate, and other foods that contain caffeine before bedtime. Caffeine is a stimulant that only makes insomnia worse. Many doctors recommend avoiding caffeine after 4 PM to ensure a good night's sleep.

Warm milk is just one of many popular folk remedies people turn to for help in getting to sleep. Most have no basis in science and we do not recommend them as treatments for sleep difficulties, but the placebo effect can be strong and if you believe it will work, often it does. Some of the more interesting folk remedies for insomnia include the following:

- **A jar of yellow onions on the bed stand.** If sleep doesn't come easily, open the jar and take a deep whiff of onion. Recap the jar then lie back and think pleasant thoughts. Sleep should come within 15 minutes.

- **Making sure the dishes are done.** According to folklore, a pile of dirty dishes in the sink can trigger sleeplessness.

- **Eating pumpkin.** This popular gourd, when consumed at dinner, supposedly helps induce sleep.

- **Deep breathing.** Once in bed, take seven deep breaths, inhaling to the count of seven and exhaling to the count of seven. Wait about three minutes, then take seven more deep breaths, again inhaling and exhaling to a count of seven. Wait another three minutes and repeat. Sleep should come quickly.

- **Crystal therapy.** Promote sleep by holding a piece of amethyst in your hand as you lie in bed. Another

piece of the crystal in your pillow case will supposedly ward off nightmares.

**This may sound like an odd question, but can sex
before bedtime help induce sleep? My husband
says he feels quite drowsy and physically worn out
after we make love at night.**

A rousing session of passionate lovemaking can be both
physically and mentally relaxing for both parties. More
importantly, it can also stimulate the production of brain
chemicals known as endorphins, which make us feel better,
ease pain, and enhance sleep.

However, some people actually become invigorated
after sex. For them, it would probably be best to make love
in the morning or early evening—but not immediately
before bed. And if sex is an issue of difficulty or concern
between partners, it is definitely not a good idea to make
love before bedtime. The act could trigger stress and anxiety, which would only make sleeplessness worse. In cases
where sex causes more hurt than good in a relationship,
therapy may be required.

# SIX

## *Side Effects*

**FACT:** People react differently to kava the first few times they take it. Some respond strongly, while others may need to take the herb several times before they achieve the desired effect.

**FACT:** Kava is quite safe but side effects, while rare, can occur. The most common side effects include nausea and other gastrointestinal problems (usually when kava is consumed on an empty stomach), dizziness, rash, and, paradoxically, insomnia. In the vast majority of cases, these problems disappear quickly when kava use is stopped.

**FACT:** Kava is not physiologically addictive, although long-term, high-dose users can develop a psychological dependency on the herb.

**FACT:** Animal studies suggest that regular kava use will not result in a reduction in effectiveness as long as the herb is consumed in recommended doses.

**FACT:** Kava is traditionally consumed as a foul-tasting beverage, but it's also available in capsule and other forms for those who can't stomach the taste.

If human beings were machines, we would all react exactly the same to everything in our lives. We would eat the same foods, enjoy the same television programs, and respond exactly the same when we ate a particular food or took a particular drug. But we aren't machines, we are individual organisms with singular tastes and desires, and thus we react individually to everything, including medications and herbs.

It's this incredible individuality, this uniqueness of self, that has enabled us to evolve and grow as a species. Cut us open and we all look pretty much the same. But on a deeper level, we are all amazingly different—unique in personality and in our biological responses. Some of us love broccoli, others can't stand it. Some of us enjoy being around cats, others are horribly allergic to them. And some of us need only one aspirin to alleviate a headache, while others need two or three.

Such psychological and biological diversity sometimes makes it difficult to discuss an herb like kava. Throughout most of this book, we've addressed specific issues as though every person who takes kava will react to the herb in exactly the same way. But of course, that's not true. A number of general observations can be made—the majority of kava users will experience this or that—but what if you're not part of the majority? What if you don't react to kava like everyone else does? If you are outside of the norm, what should you anticipate and what should you be wary of?

In this chapter, we'll discuss the potential side effects of kava use, commonsense precautions, issues of legality, and the herb's safety and efficacy when used by seniors, pregnant women, and people with specific medical conditions.

**Friends of mine who have tried kava as a beverage say the biggest obstacle to their enjoyment is the taste. Is there any way to get around this problem?**

Many people find that they get the best results from kava when they consume it as a drink made from ground root or tincture. Sharing cups of kava with friends can be a fun and enlightening social experience. But as mentioned earlier, kava tastes terrible in this form. The degree of unpleasantness varies from person to person, although it is not uncommon for first-timers to gag on their first mouthful of pure kava. Some say it tastes like dirty socks. Others liken it to muddy water, sawdust, or worse. But to paraphrase William Shakespeare, kava by any description tastes just plain bad! Even the mouth-numbing effect that accompanies kava use does little to improve the taste of subsequent cups.

Many longtime users say that kava is an acquired pleasure and that eventually you will get used to its disgusting taste. But if you'd rather not wait, the natives of the South Pacific islands say that one or two spoonfuls of honey or other natural sweeteners can make a kava drink more palatable. They also recommend snacking on something flavorful while consuming the beverage, such as fresh fruit or cookies. And finally, don't nurse a cup of kava—drink it down in as few gulps as you can. Sipping kava only prolongs the horrible taste.

If you find that you simply can't stomach kava in this form, don't despair. The herb is also available in capsules and other forms that offer the same benefits as a kava drink but without the awful aftertaste.

**I hope to try kava for the first time very soon. Does everyone react to the herb the same way the first time they take it?**

No. As with any herb, people react quite differently the first time they take kava, whether it's as a beverage or in capsule form. Some first-time users react quite strongly to the herb, while others experience only mild benefits and a few feel nothing at all. If you are part of the latter group, don't give up. It is not uncommon for people to have to take kava two or three times before they really start to feel calm and relaxed, and even longer to achieve maximum effectiveness.

There are a number of reasons for this disparity of reaction, including the form and strength of the kava you are using, how it was processed, where it's from and your own health and constitution. Some people are just naturally more sensitive and react strongly to the smallest dose of any herb or medication. Others have very strong systems that require higher doses and more frequent use. But once you start to feel the effects of kava, you should react similarly with every use.

"I tried kava four times before I got anything out of it," notes Alex, a 29-year-old waiter whose work is often quite stressful. "After the third try, I just figured kava wasn't for me, that I had one of those systems that just wouldn't react to it. But my girlfriend suggested I take a stronger dose just to be sure, and that's what finally worked. I just wasn't taking enough to do any good. I started to experiment with doses and now I know exactly how much to take to ease anxiety and help me sleep. Don't be afraid of the trial and error."

It also helps to try kava in various forms. Some people find they get the greatest benefits from kava capsules, while others prefer tea made from dried kava root or a liquid tincture. So if one form doesn't work, try another. You can also experiment with various products. Kavalactone levels can vary dramatically from one company to another, and if you find that nothing is happening, it could be that the product you are using is on the weak end.

Of course, if nothing happens despite brand and form, you may have one of those very unique systems that simply doesn't react to kava. If you're taking kava to help reduce stress and anxiety or to help you sleep but it doesn't seem to be helping, consider trying some of the other remedies discussed in Chapters 4 and 5.

## What kind of side effects, if any, can result from the use of kava?

It's easy to assume that because kava is a natural herb with a long history of use, nothing bad can ever come from consuming it. But as we have noted, people can react adversely to just about anything, no matter how innocuous; even something that seems as simple as aspirin can cause problems in sensitive individuals. This is true of kava, too.

Side effects are rare among kava users, but they can occur—especially when the herb is taken on an empty stomach, in very high doses, and for extended periods of time. But in the big picture, the side effects typically associated with kava are much milder than those that can occur from using standard psychoactive drugs such as sedatives (benzodiazepines, for example). According to various studies, including monographs from Germany's respected Commission E (an organization that approves herbs for medicinal use), the most common side effects noted among long-term, high-dose kava users include nausea and other gastrointestinal problems (usually when kava is consumed on an empty stomach), headache or dizziness, rash, insomnia, and, uncommonly, mild visual disturbances. In the vast majority of cases, these problems disappear quickly when kava use is reduced or stopped altogether and can usually be prevented by keeping kavalactone levels below 150 milligrams per day.

"I made the mistake of taking three very potent kava capsules on an empty stomach one evening and it really hit me hard," notes Kevin, a 31-year-old taxi driver who takes kava two or three times a week to chill out. "Within a few minutes my stomach started to hurt and I felt kind of nauseated. I ate a sandwich to put something in my stomach and lay down on the couch. About an hour later, I started to feel better. I learned a lesson that day—take kava only in moderation, and make sure you have food in your stomach!"

Kevin's situation illustrates a common problem among new kava users—taking too much in an attempt to boost the herb's effects, or to make it kick in faster. It is always best to start with a low dose and increase it as needed—within limits. A sudden and dramatic increase in dose is unnecessary and just asking for trouble.

Extremely heavy daily kava use can also lead to yellowing of the skin and nails and may develop into a condition known as "kava dermopathy," which is characterized by dry, scaly eruptions on the skin. The areas most commonly affected include the shins, the palms of the hands, the forearms, the soles of the feet, and the back. This condition is more common to the South Pacific islands, where kava use is considerably higher than in the United States, and it afflicts an estimated 70 percent of heavy kava drinkers. Interestingly, in that region of the world kava dermopathy was once considered a sign of royalty because only kings could afford to spend so little time working and so much time enjoying kava. Observed a member of Captain Cook's crew upon getting to know the natives of that region: "After kava drinking, the skin begins to be covered with a whitish scurf, like leprosy, which many regard as a badge of nobility the more scaly their bodies are, the more honorable it is with them."

You have to drink a lot of kava to develop kava dermopathy. Studies on Polynesians found that those with severe forms of the condition spent more than 30 hours a week drinking kava and consumed, on average, several pints of kava beverage every day.

The treatment for kava dermopathy is to reduce or discontinue kava consumption. However, researchers are still at a loss as to why the condition develops at all. Many theorize that it's an allergic response triggered by excessive kava use, while others believe it may result from photosensitivity as kavalactones build up in the skin. And a growing number speculate that it could be the result of a defect in how the body processes cholesterol.

Kava dermopathy is certainly a concern, but the chances of a casual kava drinker developing the condition are almost nil. Enormous quantities of the herb must be consumed for skin changes to occur, and most western kava users maintain their use well within safe and healthy limits.

**While researching kava on the Internet, I read that the herb can be bad for the liver and other organs. I find this hard to believe considering kava's long history of use and generally safe medical profile. Is there any truth to it?**

The report you read on the Internet probably concerned a 1988 Australian study on the effects of heavy kava consumption in the Aboriginal town of Arnhem Land, Australia. Researchers from the Menzies School of Health Research looked at 39 heavy kava users and 34 nonusers and found some striking health differences between the two groups. In the kava group, 20 were very heavy kava users, averaging about 60 grams of root powder a day; 15 were heavy users, averaging 40 grams of powder per day; and 4 were occasional users, averaging about 15 grams per day.

The researchers report that the heavy kava users were more likely to complain of poor health and suffer from kava dermopathy. Their knee reflexes were noticeably slower, they weighed less than the nonusers because of poor nutrition (in many cases, kava took the place of daily meals), and they had elevated liver enzymes, which suggests that excessive kava use over a long period of time can, indeed, cause liver damage.

While these side effects are important, it should be noted that they were the obvious result of extreme kava abuse—sometimes as much as a gallon of kava a day. Such amounts are way above the norm, and there have been no reports of similar effects in any western country in which kava is widely used.

**I suffer from numerous food allergies, so I've been reluctant to try kava. Can the herb produce an allergic reaction in sensitive individuals?**

It's rare, but there are reports of allergic reactions, most commonly in people who have consumed kava extract in large quantities. Symptoms can include skin reactions, coordination difficulties, and visual impairment. One 1985 study reported the case of a user whose pupils dilated after he consumed a high dose of kava extract, making it difficult for him to focus on objects that were close. This situation was unique because the majority of kava users report a slight improvement in visual acuity when taking normal amounts of kava.

Symptoms of allergy usually go away when users return to a lower dose. However, because of your history of food allergies, you should probably stop using the herb at the first sign of trouble.

**I'm seven months pregnant and find it increasingly difficult to get a good night's sleep. In addition, I find myself falling into occasional bouts of anxiety that are becoming increasingly common as my due date approaches. Can I safely take kava to help me through these rough periods?**

It's not a good idea. As mentioned earlier, kava is not recommended for pregnant or lactating women because of the potential risk—however small—to themselves or to their babies. There is not a great deal of clinical research regarding the issue of kava and pregnancy, but Germany's Commission E strongly advises mothers-to-be to avoid the herb unless otherwise instructed by their doctors.

Your obstetrician should be able to suggest safe and effective alternative treatments for your occasional anxiety which, by the way, is quite common among new mothers. As for your sleep difficulties, again, ask your doctor. While a number of mild herbal teas, such as those with valerian or chamomile, have a long and extensive history of use, their safety has not been established in pregnancy and they should therefore be avoided. The bottom line: If you are pregnant (or if you think you may be pregnant), consult your doctor about the safety of any medications (prescription and over-the-counter), herbs, and other dietary supplements you are taking or thinking about taking. However, if you don't want to take any supplements at all, a warm bath, a soothing massage, or a few minutes of quiet meditation may help you sleep a little better. See Chapter 3: Insomnia for additional tips on how to get a good night's sleep.

## My 10-year-old son seems to be experiencing a lot of school-related anxiety lately. Can I give him kava to calm his nerves and help him get a good night's sleep?

I would advise against it. While kava is generally considered safe, its effects on children have not been widely researched and a child's reaction to the herb is unpredictable at best. As a result, Germany's Commission E recommends not giving kava to anyone under age 18. Until herbalists have a better understanding of how kava affects young people, you're probably better off giving your son another calming herb such as valerian (assuming he does not have a history of allergies).

In some cultures, herbs have a long history of use as a therapeutic alternative for children, especially in regions where traditional medicine is still widely practiced. A mild chamomile tea, for example, is commonly used in many areas of the world to calm a young child who is cranky, colicky, or teething. However, systematic clinical studies of the effects of herbs on children have yet to be done.

But just to be safe, I would encourage you to consult with your pediatrician before placing your son on a regimen of any herb, especially if he is already taking medication regularly. Discontinue use immediately if there is any indication of an adverse reaction.

**I'm 67 years old and suffer from occasional bouts of anxiety and insomnia. I'd rather take kava than a prescription sedative, but I was wondering: Are there any special precautions for seniors?**

Not really, although I would advise you to start with a relatively low dose—perhaps 40 milligrams of kavalactones—and, if necessary, gradually increase it until you achieve the desired results. Seniors often react strongly to supplements, so it's wise to adhere to the adage "Start low, go slow." This is also true for people who are medically challenged; a body weakened by disease may react more strongly to smaller doses of a specific compound than a body that is in good health. Of course, regardless of age, if you suffer from a chronic illness or take medication on a regular basis, make sure your doctor is aware of your kava use.

"Kava's been a lifesaver for me," notes Janice, a 68-year-old retired teacher. "After menopause, I suddenly found myself feeling anxious and nervous, and I had increasing trouble getting to sleep. I would become fatigued quite early, but would wake up in the middle of the night and find it nearly impossible to get back to sleep again. My doctor gave me a prescription for a sedative, but I couldn't stand the side effects. I slept through the night, but I never really felt rested.

"Then my granddaughter suggested I try kava. She said she took it to calm down after a hectic day at the office, and that it also helped her sleep. I figured I had nothing to lose, and I liked the fact that it was a natural herb with a long history of use. The first night I took it, I slept like a baby. And after a week or so, I noticed that my nervousness was almost gone. If you ask me, kava's a true miracle."

**I started taking kava a month ago and have found that it really helps me calm down after a stressful day at the office. It also enables me to get a good night's sleep when insomnia threatens, which is a pleasant side benefit. My question is: How long can I take kava? Is it safe to take every day?**

Many residents of the South Pacific islands consume kava by the cupful every evening for much of their adult lives, but most herbalists do not recommend this because of the possibility of side effects from excessive, long-term use. Although they are rare, health problems can arise from high-dose kava consumption.

The occasional use of kava appears to be completely safe, but if you're taking it every day to help relieve stress and anxiety or to help you sleep, it is probably wise to take a two- or three-week break every six months or so to give your system a chance to balance itself. During these "kava vacations," consider the wide array of other calming herbs such as valerian, hops, or passionflower to help you cope with daily stress or sleep disruptions.

**I enjoy the effects of kava and take it frequently to help me chill out after a particularly stressful day, and to help me sleep a little better. But is it possible to overdo a good thing? Can regular use of kava lead to addiction?**

There is nothing in the medical literature to suggest that kava can lead to physiological dependence or addiction. It does not affect the brain the way traditionally addictive drugs such as cocaine do, and hundreds of years of use among the South Pacific islanders suggest that normal consumption is quite safe.

However, researchers say that excessive use in high doses can potentially lead to kava abuse and a psychological dependency. While not the same as a physiological addiction, psychological dependency can make users feel as if they *must* have kava in order to relax or go to sleep.

Kava abuse has been well documented among the Aborigines of Australia, who were first introduced to the herb in the mid-1980s by Polynesian missionaries. Many Aboriginal leaders advocated kava use as a safe and healthy substitute for alcohol, which was taking a heavy toll on the Aborigine population. But in many cases, those with an addiction to alcohol simply replaced one dependency with another. The result was an epidemic of kava abuse, characterized by lethargy, apathy, loss of will, malnutrition, and general ill health.

Herbalists and researchers say that the people most at risk of developing a mental dependency on kava are those who tend to overdo whatever mood-altering substance they come in contact with whether it's alcohol, marijuana, prescription sedatives, harder drugs, or kava.

It should be noted, however, that one must consume a lot of kava to develop a mental dependency as described above. When used as directed—in moderate doses with occasional "kava breaks"—kava has not been associated with physiological dependency.

**I've become a real fan of kava over the past few months and use it on a regular basis. I know now that I don't have to worry about becoming addicted to the herb, but should I worry about side effects if I suddenly stop taking it? Is there such a thing as "kava withdrawal"?**

To date, neither clinical research nor anecdotal reports indicate withdrawal effects when kava is discontinued. Numerous studies involving the long-term use of kava have found no physiological or mental side effects when users suddenly stop taking the herb. This is, say herbalists, an important benefit of kava over prescription sedatives such as benzodiazepines, which can result in serious withdrawal symptoms among those who go cold turkey.

People who have developed a mental dependency on kava, as discussed earlier, may experience a temporary craving or need if they suddenly stop consuming the herb, but those who use it in moderation have nothing to worry about.

## Is it possible to develop a tolerance to kava as a result of long-term use? Can daily consumption render the herb ineffective?

Most likely, the answer is no. At least, that is what studies in mice have concluded. Dr. P. H. Duffield, a researcher at the University of New South Wales in Australia, was able to induce tolerance by giving mice high doses of liquid pure kava extract, although tolerance did not occur when the animals were given plain kava resin as found in most commercial kava products. Based on these findings and extrapolating them to humans, Duffield concluded that tolerance should not be a problem among individuals who consumed normal levels of kava on a regular basis, especially if they took an occasional break from the herb.

The longest period of time that human test subjects have received a daily dose of kava under clinical observation is 24 weeks. The lead researcher for that study, H. P. Volz, reported no apparent side effects and no indications of tolerance during this period. Nonetheless, extreme long-term use is not encouraged.

## Is it acceptable to mix kava with alcohol? For example, could I drink a cup of kava and follow it with a beer chaser?

Studies on this issue have so far been inconclusive. Some researchers say that alcohol can potentiate (to make more active) the effects of kava, while others report that the combination produces no ill effect at all. It should be remembered, however, that combining alcohol and sedatives—even herbal sedatives such as kava—is a bad idea. While many people may experience no ill effects from an alcohol-kava mix, those with sensitive systems may react adversely depending on factors such as the amount of alcohol and kava consumed, the percentage of kavalactones in the kava, and the person's metabolism. There is no way to predict the outcome of a kava-alcohol combination, so caution should always be used.

If you must combine kava and alcohol, make sure the quantities of each are small, avoid driving or operating heavy machinery, and stop immediately if you feel the onset of side effects or adverse reactions.

**My sex life hasn't been so hot lately. I'm often too busy or too tired to make love to my wife, and when we do find the time, I notice that my libido just isn't as strong as it used to be. I'm looking for a natural fix and was hoping that kava could be it. Can kava help boost my sex drive?**

Probably not. Kava is not traditionally known as a sex enhancer and clinical studies have uncovered no apparent influence on either the male or female libido. In addition, certain common characteristics of the herb—such as its ability to sedate and anesthetize—could, in theory, have a detrimental effect on one's desire or ability to enjoy lovemaking.

The only situation in which kava might be beneficial is if one's libido is being crippled by stress or anxiety. In a great many cases, sex therapists note, lack of desire or an inability to maintain an erection to the satisfaction of both partners is triggered by too much stress at work and at home. Office pressures, impending deadlines, and family problems can gang up on a couple to make intimacy more of a chore than a pleasure. If that is the case, then kava's ability to reduce stress and anxiety and induce a natural sense of calm can pave the way for passionate sex by eliminating these mental obstacles. Recurring sexual dysfunction, however, should probably be addressed by a qualified sex therapist.

"My wife and I are one of those couples whose sex life was saved by kava," says John, a 35-year-old computer consultant. "I was wracked with generalized anxiety from the pressures of my job, and found that my desire for sex had plummeted as a result. Luckily, my wife read a magazine article about the benefits of kava and suggested we take it together. I really didn't think it would work, but after a week my anxiety level was noticeably lower. Even my wife could tell that I was feeling better. But best of all, as my anxiety disappeared, my libido came alive again. My job is still stressful, but now I don't bring that stress into the bedroom."

**My husband has beginning-stage Parkinson's disease and would like to try kava to help him sleep. However, his doctor is against it. He says that kava could be dangerous considering my husband's medical condition. I thought kava was a safe, natural herb. How could it possibly be dangerous?**

You should listen to your husband's doctor, who is correct in recommending that your husband stay away from kava. While kava is a safe and natural herb, health problems could result if it is consumed by people with Parkinson's disease and related conditions. The reason is simple: People with Parkinson's disease need a chemical called dopamine, and kava may adversely affect dopamine receptors in the brain. The most common treatments for Parkinson's disease, such as L-dopa and selegiline, boost dopamine levels, so anyone on these medications should avoid kava just to be safe.

Diabetics should also use kava with caution. Some studies have found that kava can increase the renal excretion of sodium and chloride, which may increase the hyperglycemic and hyperuremic effects of certain glucose-elevating compounds. If you take insulin for the control of diabetes, see your doctor before starting kava.

**Is kava really legal in the United States? It seems to me that any compound that calms and reduces anxiety as effectively as kava must be a controlled substance. What's the catch?**

There is no catch. Kava is completely legal in the United States and is sold openly in grocery and health food stores nationwide. There are no government restrictions on its use or who can purchase and consume the herb. Kava holds the same legal status as chamomile, valerian, or any other healthful plant.

It should be noted, however, that those who overindulge in kava to the point of extreme drowsiness or impairment could find themselves in trouble if they drive a car or operate heavy machinery while under the influence of the herb. Utah, which has a sizable Polynesian population, was one of the first states to charge impaired kava drinkers with driving under the influence (DUI), even though the herb itself is completely legal.

According to a report in the August 5, 1996, edition of the *Deseret News* in Salt Lake City, a driver who was weaving in traffic as if drunk was pulled over by Paul Hiatt of the Utah Highway Patrol. The driver had all the appearances of being intoxicated—slurred speech, an unsteady gait—but much to Patrolman Hiatt's surprise, a breathalyser test showed no alcohol in the driver's system. Upon questioning, however, the man admitted to drinking 16 cups of kava that evening. He was charged with DUI, but his case was thrown out of court because neither a breathalyser test or a laboratory blood test showed any intoxicating substances in his system. A handful of similar cases were also thrown out of court for the same reason.

However, things may go differently for others who drink too much kava and then get behind the wheel. Realizing that kava abusers were walking free because state laboratory analysts didn't know what to look for, Patrolman Hiatt—a trained Drug Recognition Expert—finally brought in some of the herb so they would have a reference. As a result, kava abusers in Utah now face the very real possibility of jail time if they drive while under the influence of the herb. Kava is legal, but driving while impaired is not.

This should serve as a warning to everyone. Kava is perfectly safe when consumed in normal amounts, but excessive doses can impair judgement, especially in sensitive individuals. If you overindulge and find yourself drowsy or otherwise impaired, never drive or engage in other potentially dangerous activities.

**I work for the government and I'm required to take a regular urine drug test as part of my employment because of the sensitive nature of my work. Can a standard urine test detect kava? Could kava register as something else on the test, such as marijuana? I don't want to get into trouble.**

I wouldn't worry. Most urine drug tests are designed to check for common substances such as marijuana, cocaine, narcotics, and certain prescription painkillers and sedatives. A special test would have to be performed to specifically look for kava metabolites in urine (or blood), but since kava is perfectly legal, there's no reason to do so (unless, of course, you were caught driving while impaired, which is another story).

You can also stop worrying about kava accidentally causing you to test positive for an illegal substance. The chemical makeup of kava is unlike almost all of the compounds that traditional drug tests scan for, so the chances of a false-positive reading are next to nil. To the best of my knowledge, there is nothing in the medical literature of a false-positive from kava use ever occurring.

**Kava is just one of many dietary and health supplements I take on a regular basis. I know that kava is safe when taken by itself, but should I worry about adverse reactions when combining kava with other nutritional compounds?**

Your question raises an important issue in this age of mega- and polysupplementation. Increasingly, people are turning to over-the-counter vitamins, minerals, herbs, amino acids, hormones, and other compounds to give them what they believe they are lacking nutritionally, or to improve their health. In fact, it's not uncommon for some people to consume 50 or more supplements a day in an attempt to ward off disease, inhibit aging, stimulate mental alertness, or simply stay healthy. The majority of these compounds are all natural and relatively harmless, if not actually effective. But the more compounds you put into your system, the greater the risk that an adverse reaction, including supplement interactions, could result. The chances are admittedly small, but they do exist.

As for the possibility of potential problems from combining kava with other common supplements, years of anecdotal evidence suggest you have little to worry about. The greatest concern, say herbalists, is mixing kava with other sedating herbs such as valerian or hops, which could result in oversedation and other side effects at high doses. And as mentioned earlier, it's always wise to consult your doctor before combining kava with prescription sedatives such as benzodiazepines because both compounds affect brain receptors in somewhat similar ways. Small amounts of each may work well in combination, but too much could lead to serious problems. A 1996 issue of the journal *Annals of*

*Internal Medicine* contained a letter by Dr. Y. N. Singh describing the case of a 54-year-old man who was admitted to the hospital in a lethargic and disoriented state apparently as a result of mixing kava with a variety of prescription medications, including the sedative alprazolam (Xanax) and the medications cimetidine (Tagamet) and terazosin (Hytrin). He was fine the next day, but his case illustrates the potential risk of combining sedating herbs with prescription sedatives and other medications.

There is very little clinical data regarding potential interactions between kava and other nutritional supplements, so it is always possible that kava could react badly with something in a particularly sensitive individual, or if the doses of one or both compounds are too high. If you experience any problems at all, no matter how slight, discontinue one or both supplements until you have a chance to consult with your doctor.

**I admit to a strong fondness for coffee—some might say an addiction. I drink several cups each morning, and as a result I tend to feel jittery much of the day and I have trouble sleeping at night. Could kava help alleviate the side effects of my caffeine habit? I'd really hate to give up my morning coffee.**

Kava is a recognized calmative and may be very effective in relieving the irritability and nervous jitters that often accompany excessive caffeine consumption. However, there have been no clinical studies regarding this issue; all we have are anecdotal reports, and the influence of kava may vary dramatically from individual to individual.

It is probably not a good idea to take large amounts of kava simply to counter the effects of excessive caffeine consumption. The easier answer would be to gradually cut down on the amount of coffee you drink each morning until the jitters disappear and your normal sleep patterns return.

It's okay to take kava for occasional nervousness or insomnia, but you don't want to become physiologically dependent on it to counteract the effects of heavy caffeine use.

# SEVEN

## *Shopping for Kava*

*FACT:*   Kava is available in a wide array of forms, including capsules, pills, tincture, powder, and ground root. It can also be found in combination capsules with other herbal preparations.

*FACT:*   Kava has demonstrated effectiveness in numerous clinical studies, but manufacturers are prevented by law from making specific medical claims about their products because kava is an herbal supplement, not a drug. Only generalized statements about kava's potential benefits are allowed.

*FACT:*   The word "standardized" on the label of a kava product means that it contains specific concentrations of the herb's active ingredients in every dose and thus has consistency of therapeutic effect. If a product is not standardized, it's often impossible to tell how much of the product you need to achieve the desired effect.

*FACT:*   Price is not a good indicator of quality or potency when it comes to kava and other herbal supplements. Discounted off-brands often contain very small amounts of a plant's ac-tive ingredients. Similarly, just because a product costs more than all the others doesn't necessarily mean it's better.

*FACT:*     A variety of unique kava products can be purchased through mail-order via the Internet.

❦

*Betty, our midlevel corporate manager, remembers well the first time she went shopping for kava. She visited a popular health food store a few blocks from her office and found herself facing two whole shelves packed with kava products.*

*"It was pretty confusing," Betty admits. "I had done a little research on the herb so I had a general idea of what to look for, but I hadn't realized that there were so many companies offering kava products or that it came in so many different forms. There were the usual capsules and tinctures and teas made of ground root, as well as a number of products I had never even heard of before. And they all came in different doses with varying percentages of kavalactones. In addition, there were a number of combinations containing kava and other herbs, such as chamomile and valerian. I stood there for 15 minutes trying to figure it all out."*

*Betty eventually asked a store employee for some recommendations, but found that the woman knew even less about kava than she did. "I finally made my decision based on name recognition and kavalactone percentages," Betty says. "I chose standardized kava capsules and tincture manufactured by a company I knew to be reputable and that contained sufficient kavalactones to do the job. As it turned out, I had made a wise choice; the products I use work well and are moderately priced. Some friends decided to buy the least expensive products they could find and realized later that the capsules barely contained any kava at all. They have to take twice the number that I do to achieve the same effect."*

❦

Betty's story is becoming increasingly common as we plunge headlong into a natural remedy renaissance. It used to be that vitamins, minerals, herbs, and other natural compounds were used only by the health-obsessed and could be found only in tiny health food stores. But no longer. Nearly all chain drug and grocery stores now stock a dizzying array of dietary and health supplements, and manufacturers seem to be working overtime to develop new products and healthful combinations.

The result, as Betty found, is an often confusing conglomeration of items of varying use and effectiveness. It's easy to get lost amid the hype, which is why it's important to do your homework before you go shopping. Factors to consider before selecting a kava preparation or any other herbal supplement include what you want the supplement for, percentage of herb contained within the product, the manufacturer, and the price. Just because one product costs more than the others doesn't necessarily mean it's better or more effective. Similarly, you may be getting less than you bargained for by selecting the least expensive product on the shelf.

In this chapter we'll discuss what to look for when selecting kava and other herbal supplements, the various forms in which kava is available, kava combinations, and variations on kava preparation.

**If kava is so effective as a therapeutic herb, why aren't its specific medicinal benefits mentioned on the labels of kava products? Most of the products I've seen make only a generalized statement such as "beneficial for relaxation." If kava works so effectively, why not say so?**

Kava is an effective calmative and relaxant and appears to have a number of other therapeutic benefits as well, but because it is an herb and not a drug, manufacturers are prevented by law (specifically the 1994 Dietary Supplement Health and Education Act, or DSHEA) from making claims that kava helps to treat or prevent particular diseases or medical conditions. They can, however, make generalized statements about potential health benefits, and that is what you see on the packaging of most kava products, often with the disclaimer: "These statements have not been evaluated by the Food and Drug Administration. This product is not intended to diagnose, cure, or prevent any disease."

Some herbalists and supplement manufacturers balk that the DSHEA's restrictions are too severe and that the Food and Drug Administration (FDA) makes it too difficult to educate the public as to the genuine health benefits that many herbal remedies have to offer. That argument could certainly be made for kava, which has proven quite effective in a large number of clinical studies (not to mention decades of anecdotal research). But the DSHEA is necessary because it provides important protection from spurious claims by overzealous supplement manufacturers. Without such legislation, manufacturers would be able to say their products treat or cure just about anything without any scientific research to back it up.

In Germany, herbal remedies that have been proven safe and effective in clinical studies are given the stamp of approval by that nation's Commission E (an organization that approves the use of effective herbs) and sold as over-the-counter drugs. This way, consumers know that the supplements they are taking really work and that the medical community supports their use. In fact, herbal remedies are widely prescribed as a first line of treatment by doctors in Germany and throughout Europe.

A similar sanctioning board in the United States would go a long way toward ensuring the quality and efficacy of herbal supplements, as well as promoting their responsible use. A number of organizations, including the American Herbal Products Association, the European-American Phytomedicines Coalition, and the Council for

Responsible Nutrition, support such a move and are lobbying to make it a reality.

## Many of the herbal products I see on store shelves, including kava, have the word "standardized" on the label. What does this mean? Is it good?

Yes, it is very good to have the word "standardized" on the label of an herbal product. This means that it contains specific concentrations of the herb's active ingredients in every dosage unit and thus has consistency of therapeutic effect. Standardized kava products, for example, contain specific concentrations of kavalactones, say 30 percent or more per capsule. If a product is not standardized, it's often impossible to tell how much of a particular herb you're taking and how much you need to achieve the desired effect. Some products that are not standardized contain little if any of the herb on the label, although many products are not standardized only because researchers have yet to determine which active ingredients are most effective.

Indeed, standardization is essential when researching the potential benefits of a specific herbal compound. Clinical studies on kava, for example, have always used pure kava extract standardized to a specific percentage of kavalactones. That way, researchers can determine with certainty that a specific amount of kavalactones (or other active ingredients) are effective in alleviating a specific condition, such as anxiety or sleeplessness. Standardization also allows clinical studies to be repeated with accuracy. So if a study concludes that kava alleviates stress and anxiety at 150 milligrams standardized to, say, 40 percent kavalactones, you can be fairly certain that taking less than that amount will not produce the same beneficial results.

**I'm new to the whole herbal scene, but eager to clear out the synthetic medications in my medicine cabinet and replace them with more natural compounds. I understand the importance of using standardized products, but what other advice can you offer regarding the selection of an herbal supplement for the treatment of a specific condition?**

Most importantly, do your homework before rushing to the grocery or health food store. Read books and magazine articles on herbal therapies and see what additional information you can find on the Internet. Determine which compounds appear to be most effective for your particular condition and then look at potential side effects and contraindications, if any, so that you can narrow the field. Several herbs were discussed in Chapters 4 and 5 for the treatment of stress, anxiety, and sleep difficulties, but there is no one compound that is perfect for everyone. A little bit of research before you buy can ensure that you get the herb best for your needs.

It is also wise to buy your herbal supplements from reputable manufacturers that have been around for a while and are known among herb aficionados for producing quality products. Most of the bigger names in the herbal supplement field go to great lengths to ensure the quality of the raw herbs used in their supplements and have in-house laboratories and researchers to guarantee consistent quality.

If you are unsure which brand to choose, ask for recommendations from friends who use herbal products or from your doctor. Take advice from store clerks with a grain of salt, however, because very often they don't know what they're talking about or will try to sell you a high-priced product when a less expensive brand is just as good.

The truth is, price is not a particularly good indicator of quality when it comes to herbal supplements. It is usually best to stay away from very low-priced off-brands because they sometimes contain such low amounts of the active ingredient as to render them totally ineffective. At the same time, just because a product costs more than all the others does not necessarily mean it is better. Read the labels, compare amounts and percentages of active ingredients, and base your decision on what appears to be the best deal.

## Why do some herbal products contain the word "extract" and others do not? Is this something to consider when selecting an herbal supplement?

An extract is nothing more than a concentrated form of a particular herb. Extracts are usually produced when an herb contains insufficient amounts of active ingredients in its natural form to make its consumption feasible.

Extracts come in various forms, although most are made by mixing the herb with alcohol or other compounds. A concentrated residue remains when the solvent evaporates or is removed, and it is this powder that is used to make herbal pills and capsules. Most herbal teas are also made from powdered extract, but because they are water soluble they tend to be weaker than pills or capsules. Herbal tinctures, which are usually alcohol based, are often the most potent extracts available. However, they may contain up to 75 percent alcohol and should be used with caution by people with alcohol use disorders as well as by pregnant or lactating women. Tinctures can be added to hot water to make a tea or, in some cases, consumed in their straight liquid form. Make sure you read the directions before consuming a tincture straight from the bottle, however, because not all herbs can be taken that way.

## In what forms is kava commercially available?

Kava can be found in a variety of forms, including capsule, pill, tincture, powder, and root. Capsules and pills containing powdered kava extract tend to be the most popular forms of the herb—and the most readily available—because they are the easiest to use. However, many of the larger chain health food stores also carry kava tincture and root for those who want to give them a try. If your local store doesn't carry kava in these forms, ask them to special order them for you.

**Could you discuss the various forms of commercial kava in greater detail? I'm a little confused by it all, and I want to be a smart consumer when I finally go in to make my first purchase.**

Let's start with kava capsules and pills, which are being offered by a growing number of supplement manufacturers as the popularity of kava continues to skyrocket in the United States. These products come in varying strengths and standardized percentages of kavalactones, typically 30 percent or more, and are an excellent way to consume kava daily without having to suffer through the horrible taste of pure kava beverage. But make sure you do a little comparative shopping before making your choice. Kava capsules and pills may all look alike, but there can be subtle yet important differences in the amount of kavalactones and other ingredients. Predicating factors include where the root comes from, how it is processed, and how kavalactones are extracted. The most effective kavalactones come from the root, but some companies add extracts from other parts of the kava plant, such as leaves and stems, which can greatly affect kavalactone content.

Kava can often be found in capsule combination with like-acting herbs such as chamomile, hops, California poppy, valerian, and even St. John's Wort. These combinations are frequently touted as relaxation or stress-busting aids and may be effective, but be sure to read the label!

Kava tinctures are made by soaking kava root or powder in a liquid solvent, usually some form of grain alcohol, to release the active ingredients. The kavalactones do not dissolve; they stay in the solution until consumed because alcohol is also a great preservative. Like kava pills and capsules, the potency and quality of tinctures can vary greatly from manufacturer to manufacturer and is often influenced by the amount and type of alcohol used. Some tinctures contain very high levels of kavalactones, while others are more alcohol than anything else. Sometimes the label will tell you the kavalactone percentage contained in a tincture, sometimes not. As a result, it is often difficult to gauge the quality of a specific kava product. Herbalists and kava buffs note that one helpful method is to place a few drops of tincture under your tongue. A quality product, one containing effective amounts of kavalactones, will taste terrible and quickly numb your mouth. You should also begin to feel the calming effects of the herb fairly quickly as the kavalactones enter your system.

"Tincture, to me, is the best way to experience kava," states Nick, a 42-year-old security guard. "I tried pills, capsules, and herbal combinations with varying degrees of success, but I've never had a bad experience with a quality tincture. They contain high levels of kavalactones and tend to hit my system more quickly. Tinctures cost considerably more than capsules, but to me it's money well spent."

Tinctures are commonly added to water to make a beverage, although many people find the taste difficult to accept. Some users say you eventually get used to it, but others don't even want to try. One solution is to add honey or other natural sweeteners to your tea, or mix the extract with something more flavorful, such as fruit juice or Hawaiian Punch. Like the traditional kava beverage made from ground root, it is best not to nurse a tea made with kava tincture. Just take a breath and swallow it down. Unlike most beverages, you are not drinking it for the taste but for the effect. Make sure you read the directions regarding recommended dosages before consuming kava tincture because some brands can be quite potent. In most cases, a single dropperful or less is sufficient. Caution should be used by people abstaining from alcohol because tinctures may be up to 150 proof.

Kava tea has been around for a while and can usually be found in well-stocked grocery and health food stores. It should be noted, however, that most commercial kava teas are considerably less potent than kava tablets or tinctures because powdered teas must be water soluble and kava's most effective active ingredients are fat soluble. Nonetheless, many people find kava teas soothing and users simply looking to take the edge off a hard day may find them effective. Like tinctures, however, kava teas tend to be on the bitter side, so you may want to make them more palatable by adding a dollop of honey or other natural sweetener.

Kava comes in a variety of lesser known forms, too, such as kava paste and kava spray. Many such products are available only by mail order, but they do offer unique forms of administration. Kava paste is used most commonly as a numbing agent for painful teeth or gums. It looks like a dark form of toothpaste and is simply rubbed onto the sensitive area. One company, Kava Kauai, offers a unique paste the consistency of peanut butter that combines kava powder with honey. Called Bee Mellow, it's a bit more potent than most commercial powders but is substantially less bitter thanks to the honey. Some people find that the combination of flavors takes a little getting used to, but most note that it's still superior to the unpleasant taste of pure kava alone. Kava sprays are often flavored and very easy to use—just spritz it into your mouth like a breath spray. Most brands contain effective doses of kavalactones and allow users to enjoy the herb without a foul aftertaste.

**How can I figure out the specific amount of kavalactones in products made with kava extract? Is there a formula? Standardized percentages**

**don't mean much to me; I want the amount in milligrams so I'll know I'm getting my money's worth when I buy kava capsules or tincture.**

You're right, it can be a little confusing trying to figure out the exact amount of kavalactones in a particular product. However, some basic math can usually reveal the answer: Simply multiply the milligrams of kava root extract contained in each dose by the percentage of standardized kavalactones. For example, say a capsule contains 150 milligrams of kava root extract standardized to 40 percent kavalactones. Then each capsule would contain about 60 milligrams of kavalactones ($.40 \times 150 = 60$ milligrams). Of course, this formula works only if a product lists its standardized percentage of kavalactones. Some smaller brands may not. If a label does not contain this information, there is really no way of determining either the amount of kava extract or kavalactones contained in each dose.

**With all the different brands and forms of kava on the market now, it's rather hard to choose the best. Is kava better in one form than another?**

The short answer to your question is no, because the word "better" is extremely subjective. Choosing the best kind of kava product for you depends on a number of factors including your budget, your reasons for using kava, and the form you are most comfortable with. All of these concerns should be taken into consideration when choosing a kava product for the first time.

Cost can also be an important consideration when selecting kava. As noted earlier, tinctures tend to cost considerably more than capsules or pills. But many people believe that kava tinctures are more pure and thus more potent than dry powder capsules and they do not mind spending a few extra dollars for what they see as a higher quality product. Are tinctures really more effective? It depends on your tastes and your body; everyone is unique and responds to kava in different ways. A one-time comparison of tincture versus capsules will quickly answer the question for you. But keep in mind that if the percentage of kavalactones are fairly close, the effects of the two products should be almost the same.

The reason you want to take kava should also be an important consideration when you are kava shopping. Are you looking for an effective anxiety buster? Help in getting a good night's sleep? Or will you be using the herb only occasionally to help you chill out in the evening? If you plan to use the herb every day, it's probably more economical to buy capsules, which can often be found in economy-size bottles. If you plan to use kava only occasionally, however, you may want to try tincture, ground root, or a commercial kava tea, depending on your taste and budget.

Ease of use is also a big consideration for many people. Capsules are obviously the most convenient form—pop one or two in your mouth, wash them down with a glass of water, and wait for the calm to overtake you. Tinctures, powders, and commercial teas usually require some preparation, but many people enjoy the ritual that accompanies their use. Again, it's entirely up to you.

"First-time kava users should try the herb in as many different forms as they can find," says Nan, a 43-year-old editor who has used kava on and off for several years. "There is such a diversity of products on the market today that it's really difficult to judge one from the other based only on their labels. In addition, some people might find that they react better to one form than another. I prefer capsules because they're easy and effective, but a good friend of mine swears by a particular brand of tincture. I tried it once and found the taste so repulsive that I just couldn't take it again. Besides, it didn't seem to be any more potent than the capsules I was taking, so I figured why switch? But everyone's different, so a little experimentation is probably a good idea."

# I'd like to make my own kava beverage from ground root or powder just like the South Pacific islanders do. Could you offer some tips on preparation?

The more modern forms of kava, such as capsules and tincture, are great for most people, but a growing number of tried-and-true fans maintain that the best way to enjoy kava is in beverage form. That is the traditional method of consumption, and it is still the most common in the South Pacific islands where the herb originates. There are many excellent reasons for making your own kava drink. The ritual of preparation makes the drink special, and when a kava beverage is made with ground root or quality powder, it can pack a potent punch. Also, it's still the most fun way to share kava with friends.

As noted earlier in this book, the traditional method of making a kava beverage was to have children chew the root and spit the pulp into a communal bowl, to which water was added. You can still follow that method if you want to (assuming your teeth are strong and you can find raw kava root), but you'll probably have a hard time convincing your friends to join you in a bowl! If you find this too unappealing, try the following method:

1. Place approximately $1/4$ cup of ground kava root in a piece of cloth and secure. Cheesecloth or muslin work best, but any loosely-woven material, such as a small towel, is okay.

2. Place the cloth in a bowl and add about a quart of cold water.

3. Vigorously knead the root with your fingers for approximately ten minutes or until the water becomes brown and slightly frothy.

4. Pour the water into cups and drink. This provides enough beverage for up to four people. Additional batches can be made with the same bag of kava, although they will not be quite as potent as the first.

If the beverage is too bitter or foul-tasting for sensitive palates, add honey to taste. It also helps to snack on flavorful foods while drinking kava. And remember, don't nurse it; drink the kava down as quickly as you can. Your mouth may become temporarily numb, but that is perfectly normal.

Kava beverages can also be made with a blender. Combine three rounded tablespoons of kava with three cups of cold water and blend on high for about two minutes. Strain the mixture through a sieve, muslin cloth, or coffee filter and drink it down. Some kava manufacturers suggest adding a teaspoon of granular lecithin (available in most grocery and health food stores) to the mixture prior to blending to help activate the herb's active ingredients. A tablespoon of vegetable oil can be substituted if lecithin is unavailable.

If you get tired of the same old drink, try spicing it up by mixing the kava with fruit juice and pouring it over shaved ice, adding fresh fruit or fruit extract while blending, or using fresh coconut or soy milk instead of water. You're limited only by your imagination.

## Is there a difference in effect if kava is made with hot water instead of cold water?

One wouldn't think so, but longtime kava users say that hot kava tea is more relaxing than a beverage made with cold water. As a result, a cup of hot kava tea is often recommended before bedtime to bring on a restful sleep.

To make a fairly potent hot kava tea, pour one cup of boiling water over one or two heaping tablespoons of coarse ground kava root or powdered kava and let the mixture steep for about 15 minutes. Strain through a muslin cloth or coffee filter and drink.

"Hot kava tea is one of the most relaxing elixirs I've ever found," says Kim, a 33-year-old executive secretary. "I like to consume cold kava with friends because if often leads to some stimulating conversation. But when I really need a good night's sleep, I drink a cup of hot tea. I start to feel drowsy within minutes and I sleep very deeply throughout the night. I don't understand how the temperature of the water can make such a difference, but it really works for me. If you're having trouble sleeping, it's definitely worth a try."

**I live in a small town and our grocery store carries only one brand of kava capsules. They're okay, but I'd like to try a variety of different kava products. Any suggestions?**

Most stores carry the usual kava capsules and pills, but finding anything more exotic—even tincture—can sometimes be a real adventure. Realizing this, a growing number of companies have their own Internet Web sites and offer a wide range of kava products through mail order. Plugging the word "kava" into your Internet search engine should get the ball rolling, if not actually overwhelm you with potential kava sources (see Appendix A: Resources at the end of this book for recommended sites).

Two companies in particular with a reputation for providing quality kava are 'Awa Noenoe (www.mauigateway.com) and Kava Kauai (www.kauaisource.com). Both offer an interesting selection of kava products and deliver nationwide.

'Awa Noenoe offers kava powder by the pound ($26 per pound plus $3 postage) or the kilogram ($50 per kilogram plus $4.50 postage), with discounts for bulk purchases. Kava Kauai sells powdered waka kava root from the island of Vanua Levu in Fiji ($28 per pound plus postage), liquid kava extract ($10 per 1 fluid ounce dropper bottle), and a selection of more unique kava products, including Bee Mellow (a blend of pure Hawaiian honey and kava root powder) and Buzz Honey (a combination of kava, honey, guarana, bee pollen, ginkgo biloba extract, and licorice root).

Discussion of these companies should not be considered an endorsement; they're mentioned as a starting place to begin your mail-order kava search. Other companies can be found via the Internet, and it's a good idea to research all of them before placing your order. Most companies allow you to pay by credit card over a secure Internet line, or you can also do it the more traditional way.

Before buying kava through the mail, get a product catalogue or listing and check to see if it discusses the source, manufacturer, and potency of the products you are interested in, whether they are standardized, and the percentage of kavalactones contained in each. If this information isn't available in the catalogue, contact the company via e-mail, letter, or phone and ask if they have additional literature that discusses these issues.

As with anything, some kava products are better than others, and it's always smart to be a cautious consumer.

## Is standardization an absolute guarantee of quality when it comes to kava and other herbal supplements?

Not really. Herbal supplements are not regulated the way drugs are, so it is extremely difficult to guarantee consistent quality throughout the industry. Some of the more reputable dietary supplement companies offer a money-back guarantee if you are dissatisfied with their product, but that is about the best you are going to find.

As noted, a product that is standardized—and says so on the label—must contain a consistent and verifiable amount of the herb in every capsule. Companies that tout specific levels are legally required to provide those levels, although it is common knowledge that the Food and Drug Administration simply does not have the manpower to randomly confirm the claims for every herbal product on the market. As a result, some smaller, disreputable companies play fast and loose with their figures. In addition, a product that does not say it is standardized or does not list a specific amount of herb on its label has no real obligation to contain more than trace amounts, although it can still be sold as an herbal supplement.

Most supplement manufacturers try very hard to offer a quality product, but buyers should be cautious when it comes to off-brands. Because there is so little industry regulation, some fly-by-night companies take advantage of a particular herb's sudden popularity by offering their own inexpensive versions. But chances are good that the product is inexpensive because it contains little if any of that herb.

Our advice: Stick with well-known supplement manufacturers that produce fairly priced standardized products. The larger companies know the value of good publicity (as well as the devastating effects of a government investigation), so they do their best to produce quality supplements.

**With the popularity of herbs and other dietary supplements going through the roof, why don't any of the larger pharmaceutical companies jump on the bandwagon and produce their own supplements? It seems like a wise business move.**

Not necessarily, in the eyes of most pharmaceutical companies. Drugs that are developed in a pharmaceutical company's labs can be patented, which makes them a proprietary product. No one else can manufacture that compound for a specific period of time, so only the company that developed it can profit. But you cannot patent an herb; anyone can grow them, so there is little profit incentive for most pharmaceutical companies.

Things would be just as bad if not worse if herbs were to be classified as drugs or medications, because then they would have to undergo long and expensive laboratory testing for efficacy and safety before they could be approved by the Food and Drug Administration (FDA). Pharmaceutical companies usually pay for the testing of new synthetic drugs because they stand to reap the profits if the products are approved. But no company would want to pay millions of dollars to test and approve a natural herb that anyone could then grow, package, and sell. And yet, despite these concerns, the burgeoning market for herbal remedies may be too enticing for the pharmaceutical industry to dismiss. Time will tell.

**I used a particular brand of kava for several months with good results but switched to another brand because it supposedly contained the same percentage of kavalactones but cost less. However, the second brand didn't seem to work as well as the first. In fact, it sort of made me feel sickish. What should I do?**

Stop taking the new kava product immediately and consult your doctor. If your doctor says it's okay, switch back to your old brand. A continuation of side effects could mean that you're having a reaction to kava, but if they disappear and the kava seems to be working like it is supposed to, then the problem with the less expensive brand was probably one of quality control.

If that is the case, you and your doctor may want to file a complaint with the FDA. The agency can't investigate every product complaint it receives, but it will check into a specific company if enough people complain.

**What could a manufacturer do to a natural supplement like kava to make it dangerous or ineffective?**

There are a lot of areas in which problems can occur, warns the FDA. For example, a nonstandardized product could have wildly varying degrees of potency and concentration of active ingredients, or it could be contaminated with foreign substances such as other plants or even animal feces during processing. Contamination can also occur after a product has been shipped. Potency, for example, may be affected by extremes in temperature during storage or if a product has been sitting around too long. That's why you should never buy herbal supplements from so-called "dollar stores" and other deep-discount businesses; they often acquire products that are long past their expiration dates.

**I'm a little confused by some of the information I see on the labels of kava products, such as "200 milligrams kava root standardized to 30 percent kavalactones" and "1:2 fresh herb strength." Could you enlighten me?**

What you are reading are just different versions of the same information, specifically the amount of kava and/or kavalactones in a given product. Seeing this information on a label is much better than not seeing it, especially if accompanied by the words "standardized" or "standardized extract," because it gives you a good idea of how much kava you'll be consuming.

The phrase "200 milligrams of kava root standardized to 30 percent kavalactones" means that each capsule, pill, or dropperful contains 200 milligrams of kava root with a guarantee of 30 percent kavalactones, which are the herb's active ingredients. As noted earlier, you can determine the exact amount of kavalactones contained in each capsule in this example by multiplying .30 by 200 (60 milligrams).

A ratio of 1:2 fresh herb strength refers to the proportion of raw herb to base in an extract. In this case, it is one part herb to two parts base (usually grain alcohol, although some products contain a glycerin or water base). Do not confuse it with the ratio of herb to active ingredient, which is considerably higher.

**I like kava tea, but I'm concerned that I'm not getting sufficient levels of kavalactones to do any good. The brand I use doesn't have this information on the label. In fact, it doesn't say much of anything except that it will help me relax. Is there any way to determine exactly how much kavalactones are in this product?**

Not without sending it to a private laboratory for testing, which is hardly worth the effort or cost. You could also write to the manufacturer and ask for some literature, but that too sounds like a waste of time; the fact that there is no mention on the label of kava or kavalactone levels raises a red flag as to its overall quality and efficacy.

It is extremely likely that the product you have been using contains very little kava, which means you are wasting your money if you are drinking it for anything other than the flavor. The easiest thing would be to switch to a brand of tea that tells you exactly how much kava you are getting, as well as its other ingredients. And do not be surprised if you notice a striking difference between the two products.

See Appendix B: What's on the Shelves for specific information on shopping for kava.

# EIGHT

## *Your Stress-Busting Strategy*

*FACT:* The key to designing a successful health and stress-busting strategy is to determine exactly what you want to accomplish and then to create a plan of action. This often means asking yourself some hard questions. Most Americans are firmly entrenched in a lifestyle that seems okay on the surface but that is actually detrimental to their health.

*FACT:* The best kind of health and stress-busting strategy is one made in partnership with your doctor, who knows you inside and out better than anyone.

*FACT:* It's wise to prepare for your initial doctor visit in advance. For example, make a list of your biggest questions and concerns, as well as recent changes in your health or medical history. It's also helpful to jot down specific changes in lifestyle that you would like to make. This will help your doctor devise an effective health and stress-busting strategy.

*FACT:* When shopping for a new doctor, the smart consumer interviews all prospects and verifies credentials before making a decision. The majority of doctors are forthright about their background, education, clinical experience, and certification, but it's possible to lie about such things and, sadly, some doctors do.

*FACT:*    Many doctors oppose the use of herbs and other alternative treatments because they just don't know that much about them. But it's possible to turn a reluctant doctor into an ally simply by providing clinical studies confirming the effectiveness of the herbs you would like to use.

*Betty, whom we've come to know rather well over the course of this book, happily reports that while her job with the shoe manufacturer is still fairly stressful, she's handling the pressure much better than she was just a few months ago. She says kava played an important role in her gradual life change by easing her anxiety, helping her cope with stress more effectively, and gently lulling her into a good night's sleep when insomnia threatens, but it's only one small part of her multilevel stress-busting strategy.*

*What brought about such a dramatic change? "The realization one morning that I was existing, but I wasn't really living," Betty explains. "It seemed as if every waking moment was spent working or thinking about work. I was neglecting my friends and family, and most importantly, I was neglecting myself. Stress had become such a common part of my life that I didn't even think about it anymore. As a result, my health was really starting to suffer. I realized I had to do something—and fast.*

*"Switching to a more natural approach to health, which included taking kava and other herbs, was one part of a major change in lifestyle for me. I also made a conscious effort to improve my diet, exercise regularly, and just take better care of myself, all of which made me more aware of the tremendous pleasures life has to offer to those willing to accept them."*

*Betty's friends say she's like a new person. She takes an hour every evening to relax and unwind through meditation and yoga, spends as much time with family and friends as she can, vacations in fun and exotic locations (with books in her suitcase instead of corporate files), and volunteers a few hours a week at a local homeless shelter.*

*Most importantly, Betty no longer lets her job occupy every waking moment of her life. She now delegates more responsibility to her staff (something she was uncomfortable doing before), takes two-minute "stress breaks" throughout the day, and does her very best to leave any aggravating problems at the office when she walks out the door at 5 PM. "The funny part is, my job performance has actually improved as a result!" Betty says with a laugh. "Because I'm not as stressed as I used to be, I'm able to concentrate better and get more work done. My boss has commented on my improvement and even gave me a raise."*

*Betty did not accomplish all of this by herself. She was aided by her doctor, who applauded her decision to change her life and offered some healthful tips on how to meet those goals. It was Betty's doctor who suggested that Betty discard prescription sedatives in favor of calming herbs such as kava, helped her redesign her diet so that it was both tasty and nutritious, and encouraged her to exercise at least three times a week. "Interestingly, it was my doctor who also convinced me to perform some charity work in my spare time by showing me a study that found that people who help others enjoy better health," Betty says. "I decided I'd give it a try. I felt ashamed because I had become so self-absorbed that I no longer noticed those around me who were less fortunate. Now I really look forward to lending a hand at the homeless shelter. The people I've met there have become good friends, and I enjoy helping them better themselves. Little do they know that they're helping me, too."*

Betty has worked hard to develop her stress-busting strategy, and it has really paid off. Her physical and mental health have improved and she has a brighter outlook on life. Work, once the bane of her existence, is now something she actually looks forward to. Can you say that? If not, perhaps it is time you developed a health and stress-busting strategy of your own. It is not really difficult once you put your mind to it, and the effects can be far-reaching. Best of all, you do not have to do it alone. The most effective strategies are those designed with input from your doctor, family, and friends, all of whom have a vested interest in your continued good health.

In this chapter, we will discuss how to design an effective health and stress-busting strategy by going into a partnership with your doctor, how to choose a doctor if you are dissatisfied with your present one, how to set life goals that are right for you, and how to get the most out of daily stress-busting tools such as exercise, diet, and relaxation.

## Why should I ask my doctor for help in creating my stress-busting strategy? It seems like a waste of money to me. Can't I do it by myself?

A doctor is not someone you should see only when you are sick. Doctors can also help us when we are well by making sure we stay that way via healthful lifestyle changes and the practice of preventive health care. The adage "An ounce of prevention is worth a pound of cure" is absolutely correct, but too many of us never realize it until it is too late. If you wish, consider the small amount you will be spending now as an investment in your future good health.

Another reason for seeking the advice of your doctor is that few people know you inside and out as your doctor does. Most of us have been with the same doctor for years, so our doctors are well-versed in our medical histories. They know what diseases we have had, what medications we take, and what influences our general lifestyle. They are aware of the stressful issues in our lives, both at home and at work, and no doubt have a lot of helpful advice when it comes to eliminating the big problems and fine-tuning the little ones.

Health is not a one-way street, although many of us treat it that way; when we get sick, we see a doctor, who helps to make us better. But the most effective health care is a partnership, a dialogue between you and your doctor that results in optimum health and longevity. Are you eating right? Exercising enough? Working too hard? Surrounded by potential environmental hazards? Unaware of hidden stress in your life? Ignoring your emotions to the point of illness? These are the kinds of important questions that your doctor can answer. A lifetime of good health requires commitment and hard work, but your doctor can make the journey easier.

So don't ignore your doctor's advice—seek it out. Ask your doctor questions, listen, and embrace your doctor's suggestions. In doing so, you may find your life so healthful that you rarely ever get sick. And that, in a nutshell, is everyone's dream.

## When you put it like that, a partnership with one's doctor makes a lot of sense. What can I do to make this relationship work more effectively?

Plenty. Foremost, your relationship should be one of cooperation. Listen to what your doctor says, ask questions, and formulate a plan of action together. It is easy to let the doctor do all the work, but your input is important, so be vocal about what you think and how you feel.

When visiting your doctor, make sure you prepare for your visits. If necessary, make a list of questions and concerns, changes in your health or medical history, and medications you may be taking, including including prescription and over-the-counter medications, as well as dietary supplements. This will save time for both of you and will give your doctor the necessary information to help develop your personal health and stress-busting strategy.

In addition, make sure you are honest with your doctor. You should never withhold medical information because you are embarrassed or ashamed about it. How can your doctor address your concerns if you hide information? Remember: There is very little that flusters doctors—they have seen and heard it all. So make sure you tell your doctor everything. You will be the only one harmed if you do not.

Finally, act on your doctor's recommendations when it comes to stress reduction, lifestyle changes, and more healthful living. Doctors can offer advice until they're blue in the face, but advice is just words until you turn it into action. Some of your doctor's recommendations may seem difficult at first, but always remember your ultimate goal—less stress, better health, and an improved outlook on life. You may even want to write your goals down and place them where they will inspire you every day. Before you know it, you will feel like a new person.

### I was recently transferred so I'm new in town and in need of a new doctor. How do I go about selecting someone?

There are a number of ways to find a good doctor. Today so many people are in health maintenance organizations (HMOs), where they choose a doctor from a set list, that finding a doctor independently is often not an issue. However, if you do need to find a doctor, the first and most obvious way is to talk to friends and coworkers whose opinions you trust and value. Without prying, ask them if they're happy with their doctors and whether or not they would recommend them. Jot down those names that come up again and again—that will give you a short list of doctors to check out first.

Sometimes, however, friends and coworkers are not very helpful. Perhaps they have not been to a doctor in a while, or are involved in a managed care program and are uncomfortable recommending a doctor who was essentially selected for them. If this happens, don't despair; there are a number of other places to which you can turn for recommendations. They include the following:

- **Area medical referral services.** These companies often advertise on television and radio or in the telephone book and will happily give you a long list of doctors in your area. But remember: Doctors pay to be on this list, so it is not exactly an objective recommendation. Still, referral companies can usually tell you where the doctors on the list went to medical school, whether or not they are board certified, how long they have been practicing, and general office information.

- **State, county, and regional medical boards.** Some will make referrals, some will not. It can't hurt to call.

- **Area hospitals.** Many medical centers offer a referral service, which is usually comprised of doctors who have attending privileges there.

- **Friends and acquaintances who are in the medical profession, such as doctors, nurses, and technicians.** These people usually have the inside scoop on area doctors because they work closely with them and can tell you truthfully which doctors are good and which should be avoided.

The one place you should *not* look when searching for a new doctor is the Yellow Pages of the telephone book. Choosing a doctor at random, or because of a nice display ad, is an unreliable way to select the person who will be in charge of your health. The few things a doctor's listing in the Yellow Pages tells you—the doctor's specialty and address—will not really be helpful to you. Instead, do your homework and talk to as many people as you can before making your final decision.

**After talking to several people I trust, I now have a short list of recommended doctors. Should I check out their credentials before making my selection? If so, how should I go about doing that?**

It is always wise to check out the credentials of a new doctor. The majority of doctors are honest about their background, education, clinical experience, and certification, but it is possible to lie about such things and some doctors do.

State, county, and regional medical boards are a good place to start. They can usually confirm a doctor's education and board certification, if any, and some will also tell you whether or not a doctor has been sued or has been in any kind of trouble. In fact, in some states, this information is available through the Internet.

The American Medical Association, or AMA (phone: 312-464-5199; address: 515 North State St., Chicago, IL 60610), is also a good source of information on doctors. The AMA can confirm that a doctor is licensed to practice medicine in your state, where a doctor went to medical school, and whether or not a doctor is board certified in a particular specialty. But the AMA is not a perfect resource; it is a dues-paying organization and not all doctors are members.

If you wish to confirm whether a doctor really is board certified in a particular specialty, contact the American Board of Medical Specialty (ABMS) (phone: 800-776-2378; address: 47 Perimeter Center East, Suite 500, Atlanta, GA 30346). The ABMS maintains a database of doctors who have received additional training in a particular medical specialty and who have passed the required exams. The ABMS also offers its listings in a multivolume book titled *The Official ABMS Directory of Board-Certified Medical Specialists*, published by Reed Reference Publishing and available in the reference section of many libraries. See Appendix A: Resources for other helpful organizations.

A word of caution: Think twice before selecting a doctor who claims to be "board eligible." This means the doctor has received additional training in a certain specialty, but has yet to take or pass the certification exam. You are well within your rights as a potential patient to ask why. Young doctors who are fresh out of medical school may need to get a few years of practice before they can take the test, but a red flag should go up if a doctor has been "board eligible" for a long time. The doctor may simply be too busy to take the exam, which could also mean that the doctor may not have sufficient time to devote to you as a new patient, or it may mean the doctor has taken the test but not passed it.

## Should I insist that my doctor be board certified? Does board certification really mean that much?

Not being board certified does not necessarily mean a doctor is not a good clinician. Many family practitioners are not board certified in a particular specialty, yet they provide outstanding medical care. But a doctor who is board certified receives extra marks because, as mentioned earlier, it means the doctor has met a specific standard of proficiency in a particular area and passed a rigorous certification exam. If your doctor is not board certified, feel free to ask why. But keep in mind that board certification is not the final word when it comes to health care and it should not be the deciding factor in whether you want a particular doctor to take care of you. There are many other factors to consider as well including personality, education, length of practice, and positive word-of-mouth.

It is important to note that doctors who are board certified are not necessarily up-to-date in their particular specialty. Most but not all specialty boards require doctors to become recertified on a regular basis, so it is conceivable that the medical knowledge of a doctor who was certified in 1980 could be almost 20 years out of date.

In addition, not all doctors who call themselves specialists in their advertisements or in person have received additional training or certification in their specialty. Doctors can become "specialists" merely by saying that they are. Doctors from Harvard Medical School and the University of Connecticut recently investigated the credentials of all doctors who listed themselves as specialists in the Hartford, Connecticut phone book and found an astounding number of noncertified "experts." Nearly 30 percent of doctors specializing in family practice were not board certified in that specialty. Neither were 67 percent of allergy specialists, 43 percent of plastic surgeons, and 17 percent of pediatric specialists. The moral: Always confirm a doctor's qualifications and credentials before making a final decision.

### I've narrowed my list of potential doctors to three. What should I do next?

Schedule an appointment with each so you can interview them to determine which doctor is right for you. Be sure to let the office know the nature of this visit so you will be charged accordingly. Remember, doctors are people beneath their white coats, and the only way to decide who is the best for you is to talk to them. Some doctors do not like people who are obviously shopping around, but it is well within your rights to screen a doctor before making such an important decision. If a doctor really turns you off during the screening session, all you have lost is the office fee—a small price to pay for determining early on that your relationship probably would not have worked out.

After you have made an appointment with the doctors on your list, sit down and write out all of the issues that are important to you. Ask specific questions as well as some that are open-ended so you can get a good idea of how each doctor thinks, views their patients, and evaluates their patients' health care. Everyone sees the relationship they have with their doctor a little differently—some want a true partnership, while others are content to let their doctors call all the shots—and this will give you the opportunity to see if you are a good match.

Areas of discussion during this preliminary meeting should include the following.

- **Scheduling, fees, and payment.** Do you have to wait weeks just for a simple recheck? Is the doctor so busy that seeing nonemergency or walk-in patients is impossible? How long is the average office wait? Are the doctor's fees reasonable for the area of the country in which you live? Is payment required when services are rendered, or will you be billed? Does the doctor accept your insurance? These are important issues that should be discussed before anything else. Now is also a good time to ask if you will be seeing that doctor specifically or if you will be seen by other doctors within the practice. If you want to see only one doctor, make sure this is known.

- **The doctor's basic philosophy of medicine.** Do you share the same views on issues such as alternative therapies or herbalism? Is patient input encouraged? Is the doctor receptive to questions and willing to explain things in detail? If you and your doctor disagree strongly on basic philosophies, your relationship could be a rocky one.

- **The doctor's background and experience.** Where did the doctor go to medical school? Was board certification in a particular specialty granted? How long has the doctor's practice been in your area? Has the doctor practiced medicine elsewhere? Why did he decide to enter the medical profession? These may sound like very personal questions, but the answers could be a deciding factor in whether the doctor is right for you.

The preliminary meeting also offers an excellent opportunity to evaluate the doctor's office staff. Judge them as severely as you would the doctor, because you will probably be dealing with them even more. Things to note: Were they courteous and helpful when you called to make an appointment? Did they address you by name when you entered the office? How do they treat other patients in the waiting room? Do they keep you notified if there is a delay? Is the office atmosphere friendly and familiar, or cold and sullen? Office personnel who treat each other nicely will probably treat the doctor's clients in a similar fashion. The office environment should make you feel comfortable.

Donna, a 40-year-old librarian, once left a doctor because the office staff was rude and inconsiderate. "The doctor was pretty nice, but I dreaded going to the office because the doctor's staff were just horrible," she recalls. "They acted as if it was a huge imposition to answer your questions, and they were generally unpleasant to be around. I once heard two members of the staff laughing over the embarrassing details of another patient's problem, which I thought was unconscionable. I finally got up the nerve to tell the doctor how the staff was acting, but nothing changed so I left that doctor and went to another one whose office staff actually made me feel welcome and who seemed genuinely concerned about my health."

### Do I have to make an appointment with prospective doctors? Can't I just ask some questions over the telephone?

No. Most doctors are very busy and it is unfair to expect them to spend part of their time answering your questions without compensating them for it. You will probably be charged a minimal office fee (although some doctors do see prospective patients for free after regular office hours) but this is a reasonable expense and an investment in something very important—your long-term health care. You're not buying a couch, you're investigating someone who eventually may be in charge of your health care. You cannot make a decision like that over the telephone.

Similarly, once you have become a doctor's patient, it is never a good idea to seek detailed medical advice over the phone. Most doctors are very reluctant to discuss medical issues over the phone because it is difficult to make an accurate diagnosis without actually seeing the patient in person. A verbal description of a patient's symptoms may actually prove to be something else when viewed in the office.

There are also professional and legal reasons for refusing phone consultations. Minutes on the phone mean minutes away from in-office patients, many of whom may have been waiting quite a long time to see the doctor. There is also the possibility of being sued for making a wrong diagnosis. As silly as it may sound, it is a very real threat and most doctors take it seriously. It is inappropriate and potentially dangerous to offer a medical opinion to a patient the doctor has not seen, which is why most good doctors will simply say, "Make an appointment!"

**I recently shopped around for a new doctor and I thought I had found one who was compatible with my personal philosophies of health care. However, after my first visit for a sore throat, I'm not so sure I made the right decision. The doctor spent only a few minutes with me, barely talked to me at all, and I came away feeling as if I had received less than I was entitled to. Am I right to feel that something is wrong? Are there any telltale signs of a poor medical checkup?**

Absolutely—and you have already experienced one of the most common. Insufficient time with a patient is only one of a number of indications of a poor medical interview, say health care experts, but it's at the top of the Patient Complaint Hit Parade. Of course, some situations require only a few minutes of a doctor's time, but a patient should never feel rushed or that a visit is an inconvenience. You are paying for the doctor's time, and you are entitled to as much of it as you personally need (within limits, of course). A doctor who rushes frantically between examining rooms or cannot even find the time to answer a patient's basic questions is too overworked to provide adequate health care. If this happens again, you might be wise to find another doctor.

The following are other common complaints or signs of a less than adequate medical interview.

- **Poor communication skills**. Doctors are taught in medical school to listen closely to a patient's complaints and then ask follow-up questions that will help guide them toward an accurate diagnosis. But studies have found that doctors typically do not listen to what a patient is saying, interrupt frequently, and ask leading questions, a situation compounded by the constraints placed by managed health care. In short, many doctors are lousy interviewers. They also tend to speak in "medicalese" rather than in lay terms, which leaves many patients confused and frustrated. If you find your doctor acting this way, ask questions until you are sure you understand what your doctor is saying. Make it clear that you are not done talking yet. You may need to do this several times until the message gets across.

- **Disregard for or lack of interest in the patient's opinions and concerns**. Some doctors believe that because they went to medical school and you did not, your views and opinions do not mean much. Their job as the doctor is to diagnose and treat, and your job as the patient is to sit there and do what they say.

  In truth, your opinions and concerns are extremely valuable in diagnosis and treatment. After all, you know what the symptoms are and your description of them can reveal volumes about what the problem might be. However, studies have found that the majority of patients are reluctant to offer their opinion on a problem without prompting, and most doctors simply do not ask. So take the initiative and tell your doctor everything you can about your problem and your concerns—and make sure the doctor is listening. A doctor's heartfelt emotional and moral support can be as important as any medication or procedure when it comes to treating illness.

- **An unwillingness to ask embarrassing questions or address potentially sensitive issues.** Some doctors may be reluctant to bring up issues such as sex, drug use, or lifestyle because it seems inappropriate and they do not want to embarrass either themselves or their patients. However, a discussion of sexual history and lifestyle is often necessary for the accurate diagnosis of certain diseases and conditions. Doctors who steadfastly refuse to enter that arena are providing less than adequate health care and may be jeopardizing the health of their patients.

- **Failure to treat the patient with respect and kindness**. The sad truth is that some doctors, who may be stressed and overworked, may fail to pay adequate attention to their patients. In an attempt to care for as many patients as possible, some doctors may appear unnecessarily (and unintentionally) abrupt or curt. Lack of respect may be as innocent as referring to patients by their first names without permission, or as serious as inappropriate behavior during an exam.

Some doctors are genuinely unaware that their actions are perceived as disrespectful, while others simply do not care. But the issue should be brought up and corrected every time it occurs. If it appears that your doctor does not care or laughs it off, find another doctor immediately. You have a right to be treated with courtesy and respect every time you see a doctor.

**I'm starting a job in a new town and I just signed up with a new doctor. My employment requires me to have a complete physical exam, which I've never received before. How can I be sure my new doctor does a good job? The physical exam will be our first real appointment so I don't really know what to expect.**

It's good that your first appointment with your new doctor is a complete physical exam because this will provide a baseline evaluation of your general health. Most doctors understand the importance of a physical exam and do a good job, but there are some doctors who may not perform a thorough physical exam, possibly at the expense of their patient's health. Here are the signs of a good physical exam, and thus the quality of care you can expect from your new doctor:

- **The examination is thorough.** Obtaining a patient's history and performing a physical exam is not a three-minute procedure. It takes time to get a complete medical and family history, check all body systems, and take a patient's vital signs, including pulse, blood pressure, respiratory rate, and temperature. If your doctor simply listens to your heart, taps your knee, and sends you on your way, you have been cheated. A thorough history and exam should take around 20 or 30 minutes to complete, and you should be asked to change into a gown. It is difficult to perform a good physical exam through street clothes.

- **The doctor demonstrates thorough cleanliness and practices universal precautions when necessary.** Doctors see sick people all day long, and it is easy to transfer dangerous germs from one patient to another if good hygiene practices are not observed. Thoughtful (and health-conscious) doctors wash their hands before seeing a new patient, after handling examination equipment, and again after examining the patient. This may seem like common sense, but researchers at the University of Washington found that most doctors wash their hands only 26 percent as often as recommended.

Universal precautions, such as wearing gloves, should be observed when the doctor examines your mouth or other parts of the body, or when drawing blood or performing other invasive procedures. Many doctors also wear eye protection such as goggles when working with blood and other bodily fluids, just to be on the safe side. All equipment that touches a patient's body should be disinfected, and disposable items such as used syringes safely thrown away. Failure to adhere to these practices should be cause for alarm.

- **The doctor asks a lot of questions.** Doctors aren't mind readers. They can't be expected to know everything about their patients simply by peering into their ears and listening to their heart and lungs. An effective physical exam and initial interview should include a lot of questions about the patient's personal and family medical history, lifestyle, chronic health problems if any, allergies, medications the patient takes regularly or only as needed, including dietary supplements, and the patient's general health. The doctor should also ask the patient to voice any medical concerns or questions, and take the time to answer them in an understandable way. A red flag should go up if your doctor doesn't ask any questions or seems unconcerned when you bring up the issue.

**I was raised in an era where people listened to their doctors, did as they were told, and didn't raise a fuss. But my daughter says I should be a little more assertive with my doctor and take a more active role in my health care. I guess she's right, but the idea makes me uncomfortable.**

There's a big difference between being assertive and being obnoxious. Most doctors welcome input from their patients because it makes their job easier. Yet many patients, like you, are content not to question their doctors. However, it is important that you keep a close eye on your doctor and make sure that your needs are taken into consideration. Have your doctor explain the need and value for every procedure and keep you apprised every step of the way.

Sometimes this requires being a bit more assertive with your doctor. In a friendly but firm tone, tell your doctor you want to be kept informed and that you would appreciate a detailed explanation of every procedure or test that is done. The simple fact is that assertive patients usually receive better health care than those who never say a word. Some doctors become annoyed when patients take such a keen interest in their work, but most don't mind and will happily oblige. You're paying them for their services, so you have a right to know what they are doing and why. If your doctor balks at your sudden change, it might be time to find another doctor.

It is also a good idea to educate yourself regarding your body and your health. Read books on general health care and maintenance and research via available literature and the Internet any chronic conditions you might have. In addition, ask your doctor to recommend educational resources. That way, you will be able to talk intelligently with your doctor about your concerns and understand your doctor's responses a little better, as well as gaining a greater understanding of your health problems. An educated consumer is a smart consumer, and this applies to health care as much as anything else.

**I recently switched doctors because my previous one retired. My new doctor shares a practice with a nurse practitioner, and I'm told that I'll be seeing both of them. I don't want to see a nurse, I want to see a doctor! What should I do?**

Give the nurse practitioner a chance. You might find that you feel even more comfortable with a nurse practitioner than with a doctor!

More and more doctors are bringing in advanced-practice personnel such as nurse practitioners and physician assistants to handle many of the day-to-day medical problems that typically take up so much of a doctor's precious time. This not only gives the doctor more free time to address truly urgent cases, it also keeps the other clients from having to wait so long to see someone. Nurse practitioners, physician assistants, and other advanced-practice staff also help keep down the cost of medical care because their salaries are generally a lot less than that of a medical doctor (that's why health maintenance organizations, or HMOs, employ so many of them).

If you're worried about quality of care, you needn't be. Certified nurse practitioners and physician assistants have completed several years of additional medical training, so they are more than capable of meeting many of your medical needs. In many states, nurse practitioners and physician assistants are licensed to do many things a doctor does, including prescribing medication. They can perform physical exams, order certain types of tests, and interpret the results. And if they run into a problem, the doctor is right next door. Best of all, though, because nurse practitioners and physician assistants are still relatively new, most of them are very up-to-date on the latest medical information.

### Are nurse practitioners and physician assistants the same thing?

No. Their education and medical philosophies are often quite different, as is their scope of practice. Nurse practitioners usually study in a nursing school, so they tend to embrace a more holistic approach to medicine. They typically spend more time with patients and look at the whole person rather than just the ailment. Most physician assistant programs are associated with large medical schools, so the majority of their instructors are doctors. As a result, physician assistants tend to develop the same attitudes and opinions as their mentors. This is not to suggest that physician assistants aren't good clinicians—they are. It's just that they tend to look at the illness first and the whole patient second.

In addition, nurse practitioners are able to practice independently in most states, whereas physician assistants must always work under the close supervision of a medical doctor.

**I'm somewhat limited in my choice of area doctors, so I checked them all out and made the best decision I could. My doctor is pretty nice and seems to be knowledgeable, but we don't share the same philosophy regarding herbal medicine. I'm a strong believer in the benefits of herbal therapy when appropriate, whereas my doctor says all herbs are worthless. What should I do?**

Many doctors have yet to recognize the potential therapeutic value of herbs and other supplements. They were taught that the best drugs are manufactured in a laboratory, and that only peasants in Third World countries turn to herbs for the treatment of disease. Of course, that's narrow thinking, but unfortunately it is still prevalent in many areas of the United States.

You have an uphill battle ahead of you, but it is possible to change your doctor's mind. Offer reassurance that you are not challenging your doctor's medical skills or expertise, but at the same time let your doctor know that you truly believe in the medicinal value of herbs and want permission to try them when you both feel it is appropriate. This is your right and your doctor certainly can't stop you. But your goal here is to turn your doctor into an ally, so you don't want to take herbs without sharing your desire to do so first.

Many doctors oppose the therapeutic use of herbs because they simply do not know that much about them. This could be the case with your doctor. If you think it will help, bring in some clinical studies proving the benefits of herbs and other supplements such as kava, St. John's Wort, and melatonin. Tell your doctor how Germany's respected Commission E (an organization that approves the use of effective herbs) has confirmed the benefits of many herbs and approved their sale as over-the-counter treatments for a wide range of medical problems. If possible, enlist the aid of an herbalist in converting your doctor into an herbal advocate.

If, however, your doctor is adamantly opposed to the use of a specific herb, listen to the reasons why. Your doctor may be aware of a more recent study or medical report regarding adverse reactions or contraindications for the herb you propose to use. And remember, too, that herbs are not always the best treatment for every medical problem. Many times, such as with cancer and heart disease, more conventional medications should be the therapy of choice.

**You've talked about finding a doctor, but how about finding a qualified psychotherapist? Kava has helped reduce the anxiety in my life, but I still suffer from some problems that would probably benefit from psychotherapy. Any suggestions?**

Finding a good psychotherapist is quite similar to finding a good medical doctor. The same sources still apply, including friends and family, referral agencies, hospitals, counseling and support groups, and individuals in the field.

A good therapist, like a good medical doctor, can work wonders. That is why it is essential that you check out a psychotherapist's credentials before becoming a client. The psychotherapist that you choose should have training and experience treating your particular problem and should share your values and expectations. If you have contrasting philosophies on what therapy is and what it should accomplish, you will probably just end up wasting your money.

Issues to discuss on your first visit include where the therapist trained, background and credentials, philosophy of treatment, how often the therapist expects to see you, how long your treatment should last (some problems can be treated very quickly, while others may require years of treatment, such as with psychoanalysis), fees, and method of payment.

You sound like you know what you are looking for, but many people are confused about the various types of therapists. A quick review: a psychiatrist is a doctor who has successfully completed four years of medical school as well as an additional four years of psychiatric residency, including training in psychotherapy. Psychiatrists are the only psychotherapists who can prescribe medications or perform physical exams. A licensed psychologist has a graduate degree (PhD) in clinical, educational, or experimental psychology and is trained in treating emotional problems and practicing psychotherapy. A psychoanalyst (who can be either a psychologist or a psychiatrist) also has additional training in psychoanalysis.

**Now that I've finally found a doctor I like and trust, how should my doctor and I go about designing my personal lifestyle strategy? I want to conquer the stress in my life as well as develop a more healthful approach to life.**

It appears that you are already setting goals, which means you are halfway there. The key to designing your personal strategy is to determine exactly what you want to accomplish—in your case, less stress and a more healthful lifestyle—and then figure out how to do it.

This often means asking yourself some hard questions. Most Americans are firmly entrenched in a lifestyle that seems okay on the surface but that on closer examination is actually detrimental to our health. We eat all the wrong foods, smoke tobacco, drink too much alcohol and caffeine, exercise inadequately if at all, and unwittingly revel in the stressfulness of life.

A more healthful and less stressful life means making some important sacrifices and being able to say "no." But it doesn't have to be all drudgery. Many important lifestyle changes are simply a matter of selecting one thing over another. Skinless chicken instead of a fatty steak. Walking to the neighborhood grocery instead of taking the car. Asking for a transfer within your company rather than suffering the unrelenting stress of your current position. What we are talking about here is breaking old habits and establishing better, more healthful ones. And that is not as difficult as you may think.

As you set your goals, be wary of naysayers—people who do not want you to change or tell you that you'll never make it. Some people often have their own agenda (they may feel they will be losing a beer-drinking buddy or fellow couch potato) or—particularly if they are family members—they may be wary of the effect that the changes you are making will have on them. Children may be especially sensitive to changes that you make, and may complain about your new cuisine and emphasis on exercise until you start to believe it would just be easier to give in. Explain the benefits of your new lifestyle. And encourage them to help by letting them choose their own healthful menu and athletic activities. Pretty soon the whole family will be living and feeling better.

As stated earlier, designing your strategy should be a collaboration with your doctor, whose input and advice you should solicit and follow. Let your doctor explain to your children why you are making such big changes (sometimes things make more sense when they come from an "expert" rather than Mom and Dad). And stay in contact with your doctor as you put your plan into action; keep your doctor apprised of your progress (as well as any changes in your medical history) and schedule a follow-up visit every six months or so. No plan is perfect from the onset; most need to be fine-tuned a little along the way.

What should your goals be? That depends entirely on you. Everyone's needs are different. Some people eat well, but don't exercise at all. Others eat nothing but junk food, but spend hours a week at the gym. And many eat well and exercise regularly but are constantly ill because of the stress in their lives.

Take stock of your current situation, and be honest with yourself. Mowing the lawn every other Saturday doesn't count as regular exercise, just as eating broiled chicken once a month doesn't count as a healthful diet. If necessary, make a list of what is wrong with your life and the changes you would like to make. Talk with your spouse and family to determine what you really want to accomplish—then figure out how you can do it. For many people, that is the most difficult aspect of this plan. They know what's wrong; they just don't want to change it. They like their lousy diet and sedentary lifestyle and two-pack-a-day cigarette habit. It feels comfortable to them. But deep down, they also know it is killing them.

You may be in partnership with your doctor, but ultimately the success of your strategy depends solely on you. No amount of pushing and prodding by your doctor can make you change unless you really want to.

"My wife and I actually wrote out a contract," notes Leonard, a 44-year-old civil engineer. "We drew up a lengthy list of the lifestyle changes we wanted to make and then talked with our doctor to develop a sure-fire game plan. For example, we now make a weekly menu and stick to it to make sure we're eating properly. And we joined a gym and we spot each other while exercising. Individually, we probably would have lasted less than a week before falling back into our old habits, but by working together we keep each other motivated. And every week, we're finding it easier and easier to reach our goals."

**I've been told that one of the keys to a more healthful lifestyle is a strong emphasis on preventive medicine. Do you have any advice on how to incorporate this philosophy into my personal lifestyle strategy?**

The philosophy of preventive medicine places more of an emphasis on staying well than treating illness, and it is not that difficult to incorporate into your daily routine. The following are a few helpful tips.

- **Take a close look at your personal habits and change those that have an adverse effect on your health.** Many bad habits are fairly obvious, such as smoking, drinking too much, or munching pork rinds on the couch every evening while your treadmill gathers dust in the basement. Others may not be quite so apparent, such as the level of stress in your life or the physical impact of your emotions. The good news is that all of these can be corrected for the better, and the time to start is now. (If you need reasons to get motivated, consider: 400,000 people die each year as a direct result of tobacco use, and another 300,000 die due to poor diet and a lack of exercise.)

- **Make sure your vaccinations are up-to-date.** Preventive vaccines are not only for children—adults need them, too. You should receive a tetanus and diphtheria booster every ten years, a single pneumonia vaccine at age 65, and a flu shot every year if you are 65 or older. Follow this regimen and you will protect yourself from diseases that kill tens of thousands of people every year.

- **Take advantage of screening tests for treatable diseases.** This includes regular mammograms and Papanicolaou (Pap) smears for women, prostate exams for men, and cholesterol and blood pressure screenings for everyone. Medical problems detected early via screening tests are usually easier to treat than those diagnosed after symptoms become apparent, so make sure your doctor gives you all of the screening exams that are appropriate for you. In addition, women should manually examine their breasts every month and men should manually examine their testicles (talk to your doctor if you do not know how). Consult your doctor immediately if you find any suspicious lumps or other irregularities.

- **Accident-proof your home.** Too many injuries are the result of preventable household accidents. Accident-proof your home by making sure stairs are sufficiently lighted and have secure handrails, bathtubs and showers are fitted with nonskid strips (and handrails for those who need them), throw rugs do not slip and slide, and nothing is left lying around where it could trip someone. In addition, make sure your home has a sufficient number of working smoke detectors, and that everyone in the house knows what to do in case of a fire or other emergency. Planning saves lives.

**My doctor and I both agree that I need more exercise. But I work hard all day and come home so exhausted that all I want to do is watch a little television and crawl into bed. How can I fit regular exercise into my busy schedule?**

You've touched on a very common problem: Americans realize the need and value of regular exercise yet cannot seem to fit it into their hectic lives. However, it is really not that difficult. One solution is to join a neighborhood gym or fitness center. Spending the money for a membership gives you added incentive to go there regularly, and most gyms accommodate hard workers such as yourself with early morning and late evening hours. Many larger fitness centers also have personal trainers who, for a separate fee, will work with you to ensure that you are getting the kind of workout that is best for you.

If the idea of a fitness center doesn't appeal to you, try getting up a little earlier in the morning and working out at home before you get ready to go to work. A brisk walk around the block followed by some calisthenics before breakfast can keep you in shape without interfering too much with your busy schedule. Morning exercise can also improve your work performance by stimulating the flow of blood and oxygen throughout your body. Another alternative is to exercise when you get home from work, preferably before dinner. Just remember to work out several hours before you go to bed or you may find yourself too wound up to sleep.

Many people quickly lapse into old habits because they don't like exercising alone. They become easily bored and grow to dislike their exercise regimen. If that sounds like you, find an exercise buddy—someone who shares your enthusiasm for a particular sport or activity and who you can count on to get you out of the house on a regular basis. It could be your spouse, a neighbor, a good friend, or a coworker. Having someone to talk with while exercising can make the time fly by.

Of course, it's important that you engage in an activity you enjoy. A lot of people spend big bucks on step machines and treadmills only to stuff them in the closet a week later because they became bored. If you are a people person who enjoys group activities, join a softball or tennis league, or perhaps a walking club. If you prefer to exercise by yourself at home, make sure it's an activity you really like and will stick with.

**I try to eat with nutrition in mind, but sometimes it isn't easy. How important is diet, really, when it comes to good health?**

Probably more important than you realize. Food is more than just fuel for your body, it can also prevent or treat a wide range of medical conditions ranging from heart disease and stroke to cancer and birth defects. But you must eat the right kinds of foods, and the average American diet seldom includes sufficient quantities. That is why so many people must also take multivitamin supplements.

Remember learning about the Four Basic Food Groups in school? Meat was the centerpiece of that chart because it was believed at the time that we needed large amounts of protein. However, opinions on nutrition have changed dramatically over the past decade. In 1992 the US Department of Agriculture (USDA) released an updated Food Guide Pyramid which features bread, cereal, rice, and pasta as its base, topped by the vegetable group; the fruit group; the milk, yogurt, and cheese group; the meat, poultry, fish, dry beans, eggs, and nuts group and, at the top and in the smallest quantities, the fats, oils, and sweets group.

According to government nutrition experts, about 60 percent of our food calories ("fuel") should be carbohydrates (bread, rice, pasta, fruits, and vegetables), 30 percent fat (including 10 percent saturated fat), and 10 percent protein. However, most Americans still consume too much fat and protein and not enough fruits and vegetables. The USDA recommends 6 to 11 servings of bread, cereal, rice, and pasta each day; 3 to 5 servings of vegetables; 2 to 4 servings of fruit; 2 to 3 servings of milk, yogurt, and cheese and 2 to 3 servings of meat, poultry, fish, dry beans, eggs, and nuts.

Of course, this does not mean you have to have every single one of the foods listed, but you should make a serious attempt to restructure your diet so that you are getting more of the good stuff and less of those foods known to cause health problems. If you are worried about culinary boredom, buy a cookbook that offers a variety of unique and tasty recipes for healthful foods such as vegetables, fish, and poultry.

**I just found out I'm pregnant and I want to make sure my diet is as good for my baby as it is for me. Could you offer some tips on eating right for two?**

Not too long ago it was believed that a mother's regular diet was sufficient to ensure her good health and that of her unborn child. But more recent research has concluded that pregnant women have special dietary requirements and may need to adjust their eating habits accordingly. In addition to helping a baby grow and develop properly, a healthful diet can also make pregnancy easier for the mother by giving her extra energy and boosting her immune system.

During pregnancy, a woman should make sure that her diet contains plenty of the following components of good nutrition.

- **Protein.** Pregnancy increases a woman's protein requirements, although there is some debate as to how much is enough. One safe rule of thumb is 50 grams of protein a day during the first trimester and 60 grams a day for the remainder of your pregnancy. Good protein sources include beans, grains, meat, poultry, milk, tofu, yogurt, and cheese.

- **Carbohydrates.** These are the main sources of energy for a developing baby and they also enable a mother's body to use protein better. Excellent sources include whole-grain breads, rice, pasta, cereal, fruit, and vegetables.

- **Vitamins and minerals.** These are the building blocks of nutrition and essential to the good health of a new mother and her unborn baby. A healthful diet rich in the right foods should provide adequate levels of vitamins and minerals, but many pregnant women also take supplements just to be safe. There is nothing wrong with taking multivitamin tablets, particularly prenatal vitamins, but beware of taking too much because megadosing can be dangerous. If you are unsure, consult your doctor.

- **Iron.** Extra iron is important during pregnancy because the unborn baby draws on its mother's reserves while in the womb. Most prenatal dietary supplements contain plenty of iron, but you can also boost your levels by eating iron-rich foods and drinking orange juice when taking an iron supplement. The reason: Vitamin C helps the body absorb this crucial mineral. Avoid taking iron with milk, however, because milk inhibits iron absorption.

- **Folic acid.** Also known as folate or folacin, this vitamin plays an important role in preventing certain kinds of birth defects. Studies have found that insufficient levels of folic acid during the first four weeks or so of pregnancy can result in neural tube defects in the fetus, including spina bifida. Folic acid is so important during pregnancy that many products, such as bread, are now fortified with the nutrient. Other good sources include green vegetables, orange juice, soybeans, cauliflower, and whole-wheat bread. In fact, if you are trying to conceive, it is wise to consult with your doctor and begin folic acid supplements prior to pregnancy.

- **Calcium.** Pregnant women should keep a close eye on their calcium intake because their unborn baby will draw heavily on their body's reserves for bone growth and development. In fact, by week 25 of pregnancy, a woman's calcium requirements nearly double. Milk is an excellent source of calcium as are broccoli, green leafy vegetables such as spinach, legumes such as soybeans and pinto beans, and certain kinds of fish such as salmon. In addition, make sure you are getting sufficient amounts of vitamin D, which the body needs for proper calcium absorption.

Items to avoid during pregnancy include alcohol (it can result in fetal alcohol syndrome), caffeine, tobacco, and illicit drugs. It is best to avoid most over-the-counter medications, prescription medications, and herbs (including kava) during pregnancy, too. If you have any questions, consult your doctor.

## I'm a 49-year-old woman undergoing menopause. Should I make any changes in my diet as a result?

It depends. If you are already eating a healthy, balanced diet, you may have to make only a few small additions to compensate for the physical changes your body is going through. But if, like most Americans, you have survived primarily on fast food, frozen pizzas, and processed microwave dinners, you may have to reevaluate your entire eating regimen.

Your body goes through a lot during menopause, but a proper diet can make things easier by alleviating certain emotional and physical symptoms, such as hot flashes and mood swings. Diet can also help you adjust to age-related physical changes such as bone loss and weight gain. The following are some helpful dietary tips for menopausal and postmenopausal women.

- **Reduce your fat consumption.** Too much dietary fat can greatly increase a woman's risk of heart disease and other medical problems.

- **Increase your calcium consumption.** This will help compensate for the bone loss that typically accompanies menopause.

- **Exercise regularly.** In addition to benefiting your heart and lungs, regular exercise helps keep bones strong.

- **Increase your consumption of fruits and vegetables.** They supply essential vitamins and minerals, and help to protect the body from certain kinds of cancer. The best fruits and vegetables are those rich in vitamin A or betacarotene such as citrus fruits, cantaloupe, carrots, tomatoes, broccoli, and green leafy vegetables.

- **Reduce your intake of salt, caffeine, sugar, and alcohol.** This is good advice for anyone, but it is especially important to postmenopausal women. These compounds can increase a woman's risk of disease and inhibit the absorption of essential nutrients.

**I'm getting on in years and find that I'm forced to take an increasing number of medications for various medical complaints. Should I worry about food and drug interactions?**

It's always a good idea to be careful and aware of potential interactions when taking multiple medications. Studies have found that seniors who take multiple medications are some of the most at risk for potentially dangerous food and drug interactions. Also at risk are heavy drinkers with liver or kidney problems, people who do not eat a balanced diet, and individuals on a special or restricted diet.

Many food and drug interactions are minor (the most common concern is reduced efficacy of the medication), but there are a few that can be quite serious. For example, combining potassium-rich foods with diuretic compounds such as amiloride (Moduretic) or triamterene (Dyazide) can result in potentially toxic levels of potassium. Mixing concentrated grapefruit juice with calcium channel blockers such as felodipine (Plendil) can cause dangerously high levels of the drug's active ingredient, resulting in heart rhythm disorders. And consuming alcohol while taking insulin can cause a worsening of low blood sugar, known medically as hypoglycemia.

Some medications are especially prone to potentially dangerous food and drug interactions. Make sure you discuss this issue with your doctor every time you receive a new prescription. If necessary, have your doctor write down how the medication should be taken and what foods should be avoided while you are on it.

**My job keeps me on the go so I eat out a lot, usually at fast-food restaurants. I know that a constant diet of fast food isn't healthful, but how much is acceptable? It would be very difficult for me to grab a quick meal elsewhere.**

Eating at fast-food restaurants does not have to mean eating poorly. Obviously certain items should be avoided, such as double cheeseburgers topped with bacon, but most fast-food chains now offer more nutritious fare, including low-fat and low-sodium meals, salads, grilled chicken sandwiches, and baked potatoes.

The real key to eating well in a fast-food restaurant is what toppings you put on your healthful choices. If you hit the salad bar, stay away from fatty salad dressings and high-fat items such as potato salad, bacon bits, and vegetables marinated in oil. Eat your salad plain, or with vinegar and oil dressing. If you like chicken, order it without skin, and broiled rather than fried. And if baked potatoes are your favorite, don't pile them high with sour cream, butter, and bacon bits. Just enough butter for flavor is sufficient—and a lot better for you.

Of course, a hamburger and french fries now and then won't kill you. But as you said, it's best not to make a habit out of it.

**Part of my stress-busting, life-improving strategy is to relax more, which is easier said than done. What can I do to make relaxation a regular part of my daily routine?**

For some people, relaxation is as simple as stretching out on the couch in front of the television or losing themselves in a good book. But others, especially those who are highly stressed, may find a true state of relaxation elusive. Part of the problem may be physical, but most of the time it's our brains that keep our bodies from unwinding the way we would like.

If that is the case, you need to ask yourself why you can't relax. Are you worrying too much? Plagued by problems at work or at home? Any outside problems that keep your brain in overdrive will automatically keep you from relaxing; it is just the nature of the mind-body connection. If this is the case, make a list of the issues that seem to be bothering you the most, then make another list of what you must do to correct those problems. Make a third list of those problems over which you have no control, then wad it up and throw it in the garbage can. This act signifies to your subconscious your refusal to worry about things you cannot fix, and it should help clear your mind. Once that is done, restful relaxation should be a little easier to achieve.

Sometimes, however, the physical manifestations of stress keep us uptight and in pain. If you come home from work every day with a low-grade headache or muscle tightness in your back, treat yourself to a special "relaxation hour." Take a hot shower or bath, then ask your partner to give you a gentle massage, paying particular attention to your shoulders and neck. Play some soothing music in the background, and keep your mind free of worries and problems. Your goal is to quiet both mind and body and thus enter a satisfying state of relaxation.

Also beneficial in achieving this goal are regular exercise (physical activity can stimulate the release of relaxing brain chemicals known as endorphins), aromatherapy through the use of calming scented herbal baths and massage oils, and regular getaway vacations with your partner. And of course, do not forget to try kava and other relaxing herbs. Taken in the evening, they can help alleviate stress and anxiety and induce a sense of relaxation that later leads to drowsiness, a very sound sleep, and a fresh start in the morning.

# Appendix A

## Resources

### Names and Addresses of Organizations

Alcoholics Anonymous
P.O. Box 459
Grand Central Station
New York, NY 10163
Phone: (212) 870-3400

American Association of Acupuncture and Oriental
  Medicine
433 Front Street
Catasauqua, PA 18032
Phone: (610) 266-1433

American Association of Naturopathic Physicians
601 Valley Street, #105
Seattle, WA 98109
Phone: (206) 298-0126; $5 for referral directory

American Board of Medical Specialty
47 Perimeter Center East, Suite 500
Atlanta, GA 30346
Phone: (800) 776-2378

American Botanical Council
P.O. Box 144345
Austin, TX 78714
Phone: (512) 926-4900

American College for Advancement in Medicine
23121 Verdugo Drive, Suite 204
Laguna Hills, CA 92653
Phone: (800) 532-3688

American Foundation for Alternative Health Care
25 Landfield Avenue
Monticello, NY 12701
Phone: (914) 794-8181

American Foundation of Traditional Chinese Medicine
505 Beach Street
San Francisco, CA 94133
Phone: (415) 776-0502

American Herb Association
P.O. Box 1673
Nevada City, CA 95959

American Herbalists Guild
P.O. Box 1683
Soquel, CA 95073

American Holistic Medical Association and American
   Holistic Nurses Association
4101 Lake Boone Trail, Suite 201
Raleigh, NC 27607
Phone: (919) 787-5146

American Medical Association
515 N. State Street
Chicago, IL 60610
Phone: (312) 464-5199

American Psychiatric Association
1400 K Street NW
Washington, DC 20005
Phone: (202) 682-6142

American Psychological Association
750 First Street NE
Washington, DC 20002
Phone: (202) 336-5500

American Society for Phytotherapy
P.O. Box 3679
South Pasedena, CA 91031

Anxiety Disorders Association of America
6000 Executive Boulevard, Suite 513
Rockville, MD 20852
Phone: (301) 231-9350

Ayurveda Institute
P.O. Box 23445
Albuquerque, NM 87192-1445

Chronic Fatigue Syndrome Survival Association
P.O. Box 1889
Davis, CA 95617
Phone: (530) 756-9242

Freedom From Fear
308 Seaview Avenue
Staten Island, NY 10305
Phone: (718) 351-1717

Herb Research Foundation
1007 Pearl Street, Suite 200
Boulder, CO 80302
Phone: (303) 449-2265

Institute for Traditional Medicine
201 SE Hawthorne
Portland, OR 97214
Phone: (503) 233-4907

International Association of Holistic Health Practitioners
3419 Thom Boulevard
Las Vegas, NV 89106
Phone: (702) 880-4247

National Alliance for the Mentally Ill
200 N. Glebe Road, Suite 1015
Arlington, VA 22203-3754
Phone: (800) 950-6264

National Anxiety Foundation
3135 Custer Drive
Lexington, KY 40517
Phone: (606) 272-7166

National Depressive and Manic-Depressive Association
730 N. Franklin Street, Suite 501
Chicago, IL 60619
Phone: (800) 826-3632

National Foundation for Depressive Illness
P.O. Box 2257
New York, NY 10116-2257
Phone: (800) 248-4344

National Institute of Mental Health Panic/Anxiety
   Disorder Education Program
Room 7C-02
5600 Fishers Lane
Rockville, MD 20857
Phone: (800) 647-2642 or (800) 64-PANIC

National Institute on Aging
P.O. Box 8057
Gaithersburg, MD 20898-8057
Phone: (800) 222-2225

National Mental Health Association
1021 Prince Street
Alexandria, VA 22314-2971
Phone: (703) 684-7722 or (800) 969-6642

National Organization for Seasonal Affective Disorder
P.O. Box 40190
Washington, DC 20016

National Sleep Foundation
Third Floor, PN
122 S. Robertson Blvd.
Los Angeles, CA 90048
Phone: (800) 748-8393

National Women's Health Network
514 10th Street NW
Washington, DC 20004
Phone: (202) 347-1140

Nicotine Anonymous
P.O. Box 591777
San Francisco, CA 94159-1777
Phone: (415) 750-0328

Obsessive Compulsive Disorder Foundation
P.O. Box 70
Milford, CT 06460
Phone: (203) 878-5669

Obsessive Compulsives Anonymous
P.O. Box 215
New Hyde Park, NY 11040
Phone: (516) 741-4901

Office of Alternative Medicine Information Clearinghouse
P.O. Box 8218
Silver Spring, MD 20907-8218
Phone: (toll-free) (888) 644-6226

Phobias Anonymous
P.O. Box 1180
Palm Springs, CA 92263
Phone: (760) 322-2673

## Internet Web Sites for Information on Kava, Herbalism, Stress, Anxiety, and Related Issues

Algy's Home Page—Medicinal
http://www.algy.com/herb/

Alternative Medicine Home Page
http://www.pitt.edu/~cbw/altm.html

American Botanical Council
http://www2.outer.net/herbalgram/herbalgram/indcx/html

American Herbalists Guild
http://www.healthy.com/herbalists

American Mental Health Alliance
http://www.psych.org

American Psychological Association
http://www.apa.org

Anxiety Disorders Association of America
http://www.cyberpsych.org

Ask Dr. Weil (herbalist Andrew Weil)
http://www.drweil.com

Awa Noenoe Home Page (kava supplier)
http://www.mauigateway.com/~kava

Ethnobotany Cafe Bulletin Board
http://countrylife.net/ethnobotany/main.html

Healthtouch
http://www.healthtouch.com

Health World
http://www.healthworld.com

Henrietta's Herbal Home Page
http://www.sunsite.unc.edu/herbmed

Herbs For Health
http://www.interweave.com

Herb Research Foundation
http://www.herbs.org

Hypericum (St. John's Wort)
http://www.hypericum.com

Kava Kauai (kava supplier)
http://www.kauaisource.com

Lee Kagan's Kava Site
http://www.prairienet.org/~kagan/kavabib.html

Mental Health Net
http://www.cmhc.com

National Institute of Mental Health
http://www.nimh.nih.gov

Natrol Home Page
http://www.natrol.com

Office of Alternative Medicine
http://altmed.od.nih.gov/oam

Office of Dietary Supplements
http://odp.od.nih.gov/ods

PharmInfoNet
http://pharminfo.com

Psycom.Net
http://www.psycom.net

RxList
http://www.rxlist.com

Stan Combs' Kava in Vanuatu Page
http://www.silk.net/personal/scombs/guide.html

Stress Release
http://www.stressrelease.com/strssbus.html

# Appendix B

## *What's on the Shelves*

| *Manufacturer* | *Product and/or Brand Name* |
|---|---|
| Celestial Seasonings | Tension Tamer (capsules) |
| Crystal Star Herbal Nutrition | Relax Caps (capsules) |
| Eckerd's Brand | Kava capsules |
| Enzymatic Therapy | Kava capsules |
| Enzymatic Therapy | KavaTone (60-mg capsules) |

| Kava Content | Other Ingredients | Price |
| --- | --- | --- |
| 200 mg kava standardized to 30% kavalactones | 100 mg St. John's Wort = 0.3% hypericin, chamomile, less than 1% standardized apigen | $10 for 30 capsules |
| Unspecified amount of kava | Ashwaganda root and leaf, black cohosh, skullcap, black hawthorne, hops flower, valerian root, European mistletoe leaf, wood betony leaf, lobelia leaf, oatstraw | $18 for 60 capsules |
| 150 mg of kava standardized to 30% kavalactones | | $7.29 for 50 hard capsules |
| 250 mg of kava root standardized to 30% kavalactones | | $21.95 for 60 capsules |
| 200 mg kava root extract standardized to 30% kavalactones | Oatstraw extract, pyridoxine-alpha ketoglutarate, B vitamins | $21 for 60 capsules |

| Manufacturer | Product and/or Brand Name |
| --- | --- |
| Frontier | Kava liquid tincture |
| Gaia Herbs | Kava Kava Root (liquid tincture) |
| Gaia Herbs | Kava root liquid tincture |
| Harvest of Nature | Herbal tea with kava |
| HerbPharm | Kava liquid tincture |
| Herbs Etc. | Cool Kava Complex (liquid tincture) |
| Herbs of Light | Kava liquid tincture |
| Natrol | Kavatrol (200-mg capsules) |
| Naturalife | Kava extract liquid tincture |

| Kava Content | Other Ingredients | Price |
|---|---|---|
| 500 mg/ml organic kava root extracted in 64% organic alcohol (1:2 fresh herb strength) | | $11.59 for 1 oz |
| 150 mg/ml kava-lactones in grain alcohol base; 10 drops contain 50 mg of kava | 55% ginkgo biloba extract | $31.19 for 1 oz |
| 1:1 double maceration | | $10.69 for 1 oz |
| | | $7.50 for 24 bags |
| Kava extract in base of 85–90% grain alcohol (1:1 dry herb) | | $16 for 1 oz |
| Unspecified amount of kava root | Chamomile, St. John's Wort, oatseed, passionflower, hops, skullcap, stevia leaf in base of distilled water, vegetable glycerin, and 57% grain alcohol | $9.89 for 1 oz |
| Kava extract in base of water and 60% grain alcohol | | $9.59 for 1 oz |
| 30% kavalactones | Passionflower, chamomile, hops flower, schizondra fruit | $12 for 30 capsules |
| Kava root powder in base of spring water and 45–55% grain alcohol; 1 ml = 250 mg of kava root | | $10 for 2 oz |

| Manufacturer | Product and/or Brand Name |
|---|---|
| Natural Max | Kava Max (liquid gems) |
| Nature's Answer | Alcohol-free kava liquid tincture with feverfew |
| Nature's Apothecary | Herbal Relax (tincture) |
| Nature's Fingerprint | Kava capsules |
| Nature's Fingerprint | Kava Formula (500-mg capsules) |

| Kava Content | Other Ingredients | Price |
| --- | --- | --- |
| 100 mg kava | 100 mg valerian, coconut oil, canola oil, glycerin, lecithin, vitamin E, yellow bee's wax, soybean oil, titanium dioxide, chlorophyll | $12.99 for 30 liquid gems |
| Unspecified amount of kava | "Synergistic herbs" ginkgo biloba, ginger, and yellowdoc in a base of coconut, glycerin, and triple-filtered water | $7.95 for 1 oz |
| Kava root standardized to 55% kavalactones | Passionflower, chamomile, hops, schizondra, scutellana baicalensis, hibiscus sabdariffa, oat seed, milk thistle, bupleurum chinense, glehnia litloralis, ophiopogon japonicus, dong gui, ginger, licorice, poria coccos, magnolia bark, fermented rice, fermented barley in a base of brown rice syrup, honey, natural vanilla, 18% alcohol | $18 for 4 oz |
| 500 mg kava per capsule (standardized, but not listed as such on the label) | Magnesium stearate | $12 for 100 capsules; $20 for 200 capsules |
| Unspecified amount of kava powder | Saw palmetto, pygeun bark, nettle, magnesium stearate | $7 for 30 capsules |

| Manufacturer | Product and/or Brand Name |
|---|---|
| Nature's Herbs | Power Herbs (kava capsules) |
| Nature's Plus Herbalactives | Kava capsules |
| Nature's Plus Herbalactives | Kava Kava Sublingual Spray |
| Nature's Resource | Kava capsules |
| Nature's Way | Kava capsules |
| Nature's Way | Kava liquid tincture |
| NuNaturals | Kava liquid tincture |
| Schiff | Knock-Out (capsules) |

| Kava Content | Other Ingredients | Price |
|---|---|---|
| 250 mg kava root extract standardized to 75 mg kavalactones | | $10.39 for 30 gel capsules |
| 250 mg kava standardized to 29–31% kavalactones | | $12 for 30 capsules |
| 125 mg kava standardized to 35–40% kavalactones | Natural peppermint/cinnamon flavor | $20 for 2 oz |
| 150 mg of kava standardized to 30% kavalactones | | $10.99 for 50 capsules |
| 128 mg kava standardized to 70 mg kavalactones | | $17 for 60 capsules |
| Contains kava 45–55% in base of pure grain alcohol and spring water; 1 ml = 250 mg of dry kava root | | $13 for 2 fluid oz |
| 466 mg kava in base of vegetable glycerin and 70% pure grain alcohol | | $23.29 for 60 ml bottle |
| 100 mg 2:1 kava extract | 3 mg melatonin, 100 mg valerian, 100 mg GABA, 40 mg glycine, 10 mg magnesium, 0.5 mg vitamin B-6; cellulose, maltodextrine, calcium phosphate, vegetable stearin, magnesium stearate, gum, acacia, gum tragacanth, silica | $19 for 50 capsules |

| Manufacturer | Product and/or Brand Name |
| --- | --- |
| Solaray | Kava/St. John's Wort combination (capsules) |
| Solgar | Kava capsules |
| Spring Valley | Kava capsules (460 mg each) |
| Sundown Herbs | Kava capsules (425 mg each) |
| Sundown Herbs | Kava Kava Xtra (capsules) |
| VegiLife | Kava capsules (100 mg each) |
| Yogi Tea Company | Kava Special Formula Tea |
| Zand | Kava Calm (capsules) |
| Zand | Kava liquid tincture |

| Kava Content | Other Ingredients | Price |
|---|---|---|
| 200 mg kava | 200 mg St. John's Wort | $13 for 100 capsules |
| 150 mg of kava standardized to 30% kavalactones | Vitamin C, vitamin E, betacarotene, rosemary | $14.69 for 60 capsules |
| 200 mg kava standardized to 30% kavalactones | 65 mg chamomile, 65 mg passionflower, 65 mg hops, 65 mg schizondra fruit | $8.47 for 60 capsules |
| Unspecified amount of kava | Dicalcium phosphate, gelatin, microcrystalline cellulose | $3.77 for 60 capsules |
| 250 mg of kava standardized to 30% kavalactones | Passionflower, hops, chamomile | $9.94 for 60 capsules |
| 182 mg kava extract and 60 mg kava root kavalactones | Vegetable base made standardized to 55% of carrot, broccoli, tomato, and magnesium stearate | $15 for 30 capsules |
| 20 mg kavalactones per cup | Sasparilla root, licorice root, roasted carob, cinnamon bark, cardamon seed, ginger root, barley malt, natural flavor | $4.89 for 16 bags |
| 150 mg kava root standardized to 40% kavalactones | 385 mg oatstraw, pueraria root, lemon balm, gotu kola herb, motherwort leaf, licorice root, skullcap, poria sclerotium, ginkgo biloba, ginger root | $15 for 60 capsules |
| Kava standardized to 8% kavalactones in base of distilled water and 20–24% grain alcohol | | $16.49 for 1 oz |

# Glossary

**amygdala:** a structure in the limbic system in the brain with functions associated with mood, feeling, instinct, and recent memory.

**anxiety:** apprehensive anticipation of future danger or misfortune accompanied by feelings of sadness, unhappiness, or physical symptoms of tension.

**anxiolytic:** any compound used to control anxiety.

**aromatherapy:** the use of specific fragrances to control mood or treat illness.

**biofeedback:** a technique of controlling certain emotional states, such as anxiety or stress, by training oneself with the aid of electronic equipment to modify involuntary body functions such as heart rate or blood pressure.

**cerebellum:** a part of the brain involved in the maintenance of muscle tone, balance, and synchronization of activity in groups of muscles that are under voluntary control. The cerebellum converts muscle contractions into smooth coordinated movement.

**cognitive therapy:** a form of psychotherapy with an active, directive, time-limited, and structured approach.

**depression:** a common emotional condition characterized by grief. Depression may be associated with symptoms such as insomnia, appetite changes, low energy, poor concentration, or crying spells.

**differential diagnosis:** a technique of diagnosing illness by methodically eliminating potential ailments until only the correct one remains.

**electroencephalogram:** the electronic measurement of brain activity.

**electromyograph:** a device that provides an audio and visual record of the electrical responses of muscle tissue to nerve stimulation.

**electrooculogram:** an electronic measurement of eye movement.

**endorphins:** naturally-occurring brain chemicals that have a pain-relieving effect similar to that of morphine.

**free radicals:** naturally-occurring molecular fragment believed to have a harmful effect on body cells.

**hippocampus:** a part of the brain involved in the complex physical aspects of behavior governed by emotions and instinct.

**hormone replacement therapy:** the supplementation of estrogen or other hormones following menopause.

**insomnia:** the inability to fall asleep or stay asleep throughout the night.

**mammogram:** an x-ray of the breast.

**medulla oblongata:** a part of the brainstem that is the primary pathway for nerve impulses entering and leaving the skull and that contains centers responsible for the regulation of heart and blood vessels, respiration, salivation, and swallowing.

**melatonin:** a hormone with a well-defined circadian cycle. Melatonin is secreted by the pineal gland at night and it has been noted to shift circadian rhythms, induce sleep, and lower core body temperature.

**mind-body connection:** the relationship between thought and body function.

**obsessive-compulsive disorder:** an anxiety disorder characterized by recurring rituals and ruminations that may interfere dramatically with normal functioning.

**Pap test (or smear):** the microscopic examination of cells taken from the cervix. Named after George Papanicolaou, who developed the procedure.

**periodic limb movement disorder (PLM):** a condition characterized by repetitive, unvarying limb movements that occur in sleep.

**phobia:** an irrational, persistent, or overwhelming fear of a specific thing or situation, frequently accompanied by avoidance of the feared stimulus.

**pineal gland:** a gland in the brain whose primary function is the excretion of the hormone melatonin.

**pituitary gland:** an endocrine gland located at the base of the brain that secretes primary pituitary hormones and instructs other endocrine glands to secrete their hormones.

**post-traumatic stress disorder:** an anxiety disorder characterized by the development of specific symptoms following a traumatic experience.

**restless legs syndrome (RLS):** a condition characterized by unpleasant sensations in the legs that compel individuals to move their legs and feet. These sensations are worse with prolonged sitting and resting in bed.

**selective serotonin reuptake inhibitors (SSRIs):** a type of antidepressant medication.

**serotonin:** a chemical neurotransmitter found in the brain and intestines. Serotonin has been linked to mood disorders, anxiety disorders, violence, and schizophrenia.

**stress response:** the body's physical reaction to stress, such as rapid heart rate and increased respiration.

# Bibliography

## Books

Aldrich M., Ashley R., Horowitz M. *The High Times Encyclopedia of Recreational Drugs*. New York: Stonehill Publishing Company, 1978.

Bloomfield H. H. *Healing Anxiety with Herbs*. New York: HarperCollins, 1998.

Bloomfield H. H., McWilliams P. *How to Heal Depression*. Los Angeles: Prelude Press, 1994.

Bloomfield H. H., Nordfors M., McWilliams P. *Hypericum & Depression*. Los Angeles: Prelude Press, 1996.

Braiker H. B. *The Type E Woman: How to Overcome the Stress of Being Everything to Everybody*. New York: Signet, 1986.

Brown D. *Herbal Prescriptions for Better Health*. Rocklin, CA: Prima Publishing, 1995.

Cammarata J. *A Physician's Guide to Herbal Wellness*. Chicago: Chicago Review Press, 1996.

Carlson K. J., Eisenstat S. A., Ziporyn T. *The Women's Concise Guide to Emotional Well-Being*. Cambridge: Harvard University Press, 1997.

Carper J. *The Food Pharmacy*. New York: Bantam Books, 1989.

Carper J. *Miracle Cures*. New York: HarperCollins, 1997.

Castleman M. *The Healing Herbs*. New York: Bantam Books, 1991.

Dotto L. *Losing Sleep: How Your Sleep Habits Affect Your Life*. New York: William Morrow, 1992.

Duke J. A. *The Green Pharmacy*. Emmaus, PA: Rodale Press, 1997.

Elkind D. *Ties That Stress: The New Family Imbalance*. Cambridge: Harvard University Press, 1994.

Foster S. *Herbs For Your Health*. Loveland, CO: Interweave Press, 1996.

Gold M. S. *The Good News About Panic, Anxiety, and Phobias*. New York: Bantam Books, 1990.

Green M., Keville K. *Aromatherapy: A Complete Guide to the Healing Art*. Freedom, CA: The Crossing Press, 1995.

Groves D. *Meditation for Busy People: 60 Seconds to Serenity*. Novato, CO: New World Library, 1993.

Harrisson T. *Savage Civilization*. New York: Alfred A. Knopf, 1937.

Hauri P., Linde S. *No More Sleepless Nights: The Complete Program for Ending Insomnia*. New York: John Wiley & Sons, 1991.

Hobbs C. *Handbook for Herbal Healing: A Concise Guide to Herbal Products*. Santa Cruz, CA: Botanica Press, 1994.

Hobbs C. *Stress and Natural Healing*. Loveland, CO: Interweave Press, 1997.

Hoffman D. *An Herbal Guide to Stress Relief*. Rochester, VT: Healing Arts Press, 1991.

Jovanovic-Peterson L. *A Woman Doctor's Guide to Menopause: Essential Facts and Up-To-The-Minute Information for a Woman's Change of Life.* New York: Hyperion, 1993.

Kilham C. *Kava: Medicine Hunting in Paradise.* Rochester, VT: Park Street Press, 1996.

Kirchheimer S., Maleskey G. *Energy Forever: More Than 1,000 Quick and Easy Tips and Techniques to Beat Fatigue and Turbocharge Your Life.* New York: Dell Publishing, 1997.

Korsch B. M., Harding C. *The Intelligent Patient's Guide to the Doctor-Patient Relationship.* New York: Oxford University Press, 1997.

Landau C. *The Complete Book of Menopause: Every Woman's Guide to Good Health.* New York: G. P. Putnam's Sons, 1994.

Lebot V., Merlin M., Lindstrom L. *The Pacific Elixir.* Rochester, VT: Healing Arts Press, 1997.

Lee W. H., Lee L. *The Book of Practical Aromatherapy.* New Canaan, CT: Keats Publishing Inc., 1992.

Lipman D. S. *Snoring From A to ZZZZ: Proven Cures for the Night's Worst Nuisance.* Portland, OR: Spencer Press, 1996.

Long B. C., Kahn, S. E. *Women, Work, and Coping: A Multidisciplinary Approach to Workplace Stress.* Toronto: University of Toronto Press, 1993.

Lust J. *The Herb Book.* New York: Bantam Books, 1994.

Matthews A. M. *The Seven Keys to Calm: Essential Steps for Staying Calm Under Any Circumstances.* White Salmon, WA: Pocket Press, 1997.

McCall T. B. *Examining Your Doctor: A Patient's Guide to Avoiding Harmful Medical Care.* Secaucus, NJ: Birch Lane Press, 1995.

Mills S. *Out of the Earth: The Science and Practice of Herbal Medicine*. New York: Viking/Penguin, 1992.

Mindell E. *Earl Mindell's Herb Bible*. New York: Simon & Schuster/Fireside, 1992.

Murray M. *Getting Well Naturally Series: Stress, Anxiety and Insomnia*. Rocklin, CA: Prima Publishing, 1994.

Murray M. *Natural Alternatives to Prozac*. New York: William Morrow, 1996.

Orman M. *The 14 Day Stress Cure*. Ossining, NY: Breakthrough Publications, 1991.

Pascauly R. A., Soest S. W. *Snoring and Sleep Apnea: Personal and Family Guide to Diagnosis and Treatment*. Philadelphia: Lippincott-Raven Press, 1994.

Pierpaoli W., Regelson W., Colman, C. *The Melatonin Miracle: Nature's Age-Reversing, Disease-Fighting, Sex-Enhancing Hormone*. New York: Simon & Schuster, 1995.

Polunin M., Robbins C. *The Natural Pharmacy: An Illustrated Guide to Natural Medicine*. New York: Collier Books, 1992.

Powell R. J., George-Warren H. *The Working Woman's Guide to Managing Stress*. Needham Heights, MA: Prentice Hall School, 1994.

Rector-Page L. *How to Be Your Own Herbal Pharmacist*. Sonora, CA: Healthy Healing Publications, 1991.

Reichert R. G. *Kava Kava: The Anti-Anxiety Herb that Relaxes and Sharpens the Mind*. New Canaan, CT: Keats Publishing Inc., 1997.

Reiter R. J., Robinson J. *Melatonin: Your Body's Natural Wonder Drug*. New York: Bantam Books, 1995.

Ross J. *Triumph Over Fear: A Book of Help and Hope for People With Anxiety, Panic Attacks, and Phobias*. New York: Bantam Books, 1994.

Sahelian R. *Kava: The Miracle Antianxiety Herb.* New York: St. Martin's Press, 1998.

Sapolsky R. M. *Why Zebras Don't Get Ulcers: An Updated Guide to Stress, Stress-Related Diseases, and Coping.* New York: W. H. Freeman, 1998.

Schiraldi G. R. *Conquer Anxiety, Worry and Nervous Fatigue.* Ellicott City, MD: Chevron Publishing, 1997.

Schor J. B. *The Overworked American: The Unexpected Decline of Leisure.* New York: Basic Books, 1993.

Schultes R. E, Hofmann A. *Plants of the Gods.* Rochester, VT: Healing Arts Press, 1992.

Schwartz M. A. *Listen to Me, Doctor: Taking Charge of Your Own Health Care.* Denver: MacMurray & Beck, 1995.

Sifton D. W., editor. *The PDR Family Guide to Nutrition and Health.* Montvale, NJ: Medical Economics, 1995.

Thase M. E., Loredo E. E. *St. John's Wort: Nature's Mood Booster.* New York: Avon Books, 1998.

Theroux P. *The Happy Isles of Oceania: Paddling the Pacific.* New York: Ballantine Books, 1992.

Trickett S. *Anxiety & Depression: A Natural Approach.* Berkeley: Ulysses Press, 1997.

Tyler V. *The Honest Herbal.* Binghamton, NY: Pharmaceutical Products Press, 1993.

Walji H. *Kava: Nature's Relaxant for Anxiety, Stress and Pain.* Prescott, AZ: Hohm Press, 1997.

Werbach M. *Nutritional Influences on Illness.* Third Line Press, 1996.

## Select Studies and Monographs on Kava

Almeida J.C., Grimsley E.W. Coma for the Health Food Store: Interaction between Kava and alprazolam. *Annals of Internal Medicine*, 125:940–941, 1996.

American Botanical Council. *Commission E Monograph on Kava Kava*. Austin, Texas. June 1, 1990.

American Herbal Products Association. *Kava Symposium Proceedings*. Bethesda, Maryland. 1997.

Anonymous. Kava-kava: A calming herb from the South Pacific. *Herbs for Health*, January/February 1997, 42–44.

Backhaus C., Krieglstein J. Extracts of kava (*Piper methysticum*) and its methysticin constituents protect brain tissue against ischemic damage in rodents. *European Journal of Pharmacology*, 215:265–269, 1992.

Banazak D. Anxiety disorders in elderly patients. *Journal of the American Board of Family Practice*, 10(4):280–289, 1997.

Cantor C. Kava and alcohol. Letter to the editor. *Medical Journal of Australia*, 167:560, 1997.

Cawte J. Psychoactive substances of the South Seas: Betel, kava and pituri. *Australia and New Zealand Journal of Psychiatry*, 19(1):83–87, 1985.

Davies L., et al. Effects of kava on benzodiazepine and GABA receptor binding. *European Journal of Pharmacology*, 183:558, 1990.

Duffield A.M., Jamieson D. Development of tolerance to kava in mice. *Clinical Experiments in Pharmacology and Physiology*, 18:571–578, 1991.

Duffield A. M., Lidgard R. O., Low, G. K. Analysis of the constituents of *Piper methysticum* by gas chromatography methane chemical ionization mass spectrometry: New trace constituents of kava resin. *Biomedical and Environmental Mass Spectrometry*, 13:305–313, 1986.

Duve R. N. Highlight of the chemistry and pharmacology of yaqona, *Piper methysticum. Fiji Agricultural Journal,* 38:81–84, 1976.

Foster S. Kava-kava: A gift of calm from the South Pacific. *Better Nutrition,* May 1997, 54–59.

Garner L. F., Klinger J. D. Some visual effects caused by the beverage kava. *Journal of Ethnopharmacology,* 13(3):307–311, 1985.

Gleitz J., et al. Anticonvulsive action of kavain estimated from its properties on stimulated synaptosomes and sodium channel receptor sites. *European Journal of Pharmacology,* 315:89–97, 1996.

Gleitz J., et al. Antithrombotic action of the kava pyrone kavain prepared from *Piper methysticum* on human platelets. *Planta Medica,* 63:27–30, 1997.

Gleitz J., et al. Kavain inhibits non-stereospecifically veratridine-activated Na+ channels. *Planta Medica,* 62:1133–1138, 1996.

Gleitz J., et al. (+)-Kavain inhibits veratridine-activated voltage-dependent Na+-channels in synaptosomes prepared from rat cerebral cortex. *Neuropharmacology,* 34(9):1133–1138, 1995.

Heinze H., et al. Pharmacological effects of oxazepam and kava extract in a visual search paradigm assessed with event-related potentials. *Pharmacopsychiatry,* 27:224–230, 1994.

Holm E., Staedt U., et al. The action profile of D, L-kavain: Cerebral sites and sleep-wakefulness-rhythm in animals. *Arzneimiielforschung,* 41(7):673–683, 1991.

Jamieson D., Duffield P. The antinociceptive actions of kava components in mice. *Clinical Experiments in Pharmacology and Physiology,* 17:495–507, 1990a.

Jamieson D., Duffield P. Positive interaction of ethanol and kava resin in mice. *Clinical Experiments in Pharmacology and Physiology*, 17:509–514, 1990b.

Jappe U., Franke I., et al. Sebotropic drug reaction resulting from kava-kava extract therapy: A new entity? *Journal of the American Academy of Dermatology*, 38(1):104–106, 1998.

Johnson D., Frauendor A., et al. Neurophysiological active profile and tolerance of kava extract WS 1490, a pilot study with randomized evaluation. *TW Neurologie Psychiatrie*, 6:349–354, 1991.

Jussofie A., et al. Kavapyrone enriched extract from *Piper methysticum* as modulator for the GABA binding site in different regions of rat brain. *Psychopharmacology*, 116:469–474, 1994.

Keledijian J., Duffield P., et al. Uptake into mouse brain of four compounds present in the psychoactive beverage kava. *Journal of Pharmacology Science*, 77(12):1003–1006, 1988.

Klohs M. W., Keller F. A review of the chemistry and pharmacology of the constituents of *Piper methysticum*. *Journal of Medicine, Pharmacology and Chemistry*, 1:95–103, 1963.

Kryspin-Exner, K. The effect of kavain on alcoholic patients in the withdrawal phase. *Munchner Medizinische Wochenschrift*, 116:1557–1560, 1974.

Lehmann E., et al. Efficacy of a special kava extract (*Piper methysticum*) in patients with states of anxiety, tension and excitedness of non-mental origin: a double-blind placebo-controlled study of four weeks treatment. *Phytomedicine*, 3(2):113–119, 1996.

Matthews J., et al. Effects of the heavy usage of kava on physical health: summary of a pilot survey in an aboriginal community. *Medical Journal of Australia*, 148:548–555, 1988.

Monane M. Insomnia in the elderly. *Journal of Clinical Psychiatry*, 53 suppl., 1992.

Munte T., et al. Effects of oxazepam and an extract of kava roots (*Piper methysticum*) on event-related potentials in a word recognition task. *Neuropsychobiology*, 27:46–53, 1993.

Norton S. A., Ruze P. Kava dermopathy. *Journal of the American Academy of Dermatology*, 31:93, 1994.

Ruze P. Kava-induced dermopathy: A niacin deficiency? *The Lancet*, 335:1442–1445, 1990.

Saletu B., et al. EEG-brain mapping, psychometric and psychophysiological studies on central effects of kavain-A, kava plant derivative. *Human Psychopharmacology*, 4:169–190, 1989.

Schelosky, L., Raffauf, C., et al. Kava and dopamine antagonism. *The Journal of Neurology, Neurosurgery and Psychiatry*, 58:639–640, 1995.

Seitz U., Ameri A., et al. Relaxation of evoked contractile activity of isolated guinea-pig ileum by (+/-)-kavain. *Planta Medica*, 63(4):303–306. 1997.

Seitz U., Schule A., et al. (3H)-monoamine uptake inhibition properties of kava pyrones. *Planta Medica*, 63(6):548–549, 1997.

Singh Y. N. Effects of kava on neuromuscular transmission and muscle contractility. *Journal of Ethnopharmacology*, 7:267–276, 1983.

Singh Y. N. Kava: An overview. *Journal of Ethnopharmacology*, 37:13–45, 1992.

Singh Y. N., Blumenthal M. Kava: An overview. *Herbalgram*, No. 39:34–56, 1997.

Spillane P., Fisher D., Currie B. Neurological manifestations of kava intoxication. *Medical Journal of Australia*, August 4, 1997.

Volz H. P., and Kieser M. Kava-kava extract WS 1490 versus placebo in anxiety disorders: a randomized placebo-controlled 25-week outpatient trial. *Pharmacopsychiatry* 30:1–5, 1997.

Warnecke G. Neurovegetative dystonia in the female climacteric: studies on the clinical efficacy and tolerance of kava extract WS 1490. *Fortschritte der Medizin*, 109(4):119–122, 1991.

Whistler W. A. Herbal medicine in the kingdom of Tonga. *Journal of Ethnopharmacology*, 31(3):339–372, 1991.

Whistler W.A. Traditional and herbal medicine in the Cook Islands. *Journal of Ethnopharmacology*, 13(3):239–280, 1985.

Young R. L., et al. Analysis of kava pyrones in extracts of *Piper methysticum*. *Phytochemistry*, 5:795–798, 1966.

# Index